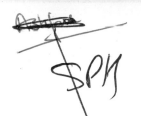

Radiology Picture Tests:

Film Viewing and Interpretation for Part I FRCR

Dedicated to:

My late father Dr. K.C. Misra.
  – R.R.M.

My late brother Maj. V. Muthanna.
  – M.C.U.

Radiology Picture Tests:
Film Viewing and Interpretation for Part I FRCR

by
Rakesh R. Misra, BSc(Hons), MBBS, FRCS, FRCR
Specialist Registrar in Radiology
St. Mary's Hospital, London

M. C. Uthappa, BSc, MBBS, FRCS, FRCR
Specialist Registrar in Radiology
St. Mary's Hospital, London

Niall Power, MB, MRCPI
Specialist Registrar
The Royal London Hospital, London

Amrish Mehta, MBBS (Lond), BSc(Hons), MRCS
Specialist Registrar
The Royal London Hospital, London

O. Chan, MBBS, FRCS, FRCR
Consultant Radiologist
The Royal London Hospital, London

Contents

Preface   vii
Acknowledgements   ix

1. Questions – Exam 1   1
   Answers – Exam 1   23

2. Questions – Exam 2   29
   Answers – Exam 2   51

3. Questions – Exam 3   57
   Answers – Exam 3   79

4. Questions – Exam 4   85
   Answers – Exam 4   107

5. Questions – Exam 5   113
   Answers – Exam 5   135

6. Questions – Exam 6   141
   Answers – Exam 6   163

7. Questions – Exam 7   169
   Answers – Exam 7   191

8. Questions – Exam 8   197
   Answers – Exam 8   219

9. Questions – Exam 9   225
   Answers – Exam 9   247

10. Questions – Exam 10   253
    Answers – Exam 10   275

Preface

The layout of the Part I FRCR film viewing examination consists of five workstations, each of four films, a total of twenty films. Each of these workstations is set out according to a 'theme' – 'plain films', 'contrast studies', 'computed tomography/mammography', 'ultrasound/nuclear medicine' and 'angiography/magnetic resonance imaging'. A total of seventy-five minutes is allowed for the examination, and information from previous candidates has highlighted how the time allowed for each examination has been very constrained. Thus we recommend that the candidate attempt each examination in the set seventy-five minutes.

The authors have set out to emulate the above system for the Part I FRCR film-viewing examination in order to provide as real an examination experience as is possible.

R.R.M.
July, 2000

Acknowledgements

We would like to thank the Department of Nuclear Medicine at Guy's Hospital London, for providing a set of varied and interesting images for use in the book.

Exam 1

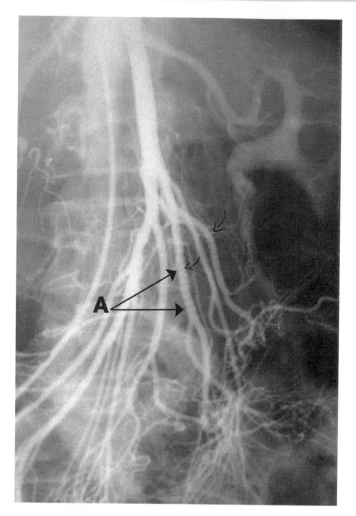

Question 1

1. What is this investigation?
2. What catheters may be used for this study?
3. What is the normal volume and rate of contrast administration?
4. What is the cause of appearance A?
5. Is this the first injection of contrast and if not, how do you know?

Exam I

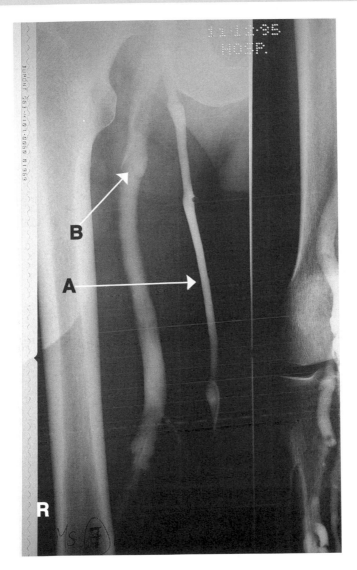

Question 2

1. What is this investigation?
2. Name structure A.
3. Name structure B.
4. Describe the type of contrast medium used for this investigation.
5. Name two alternative investigations to assess the deep veins of the lower limb.

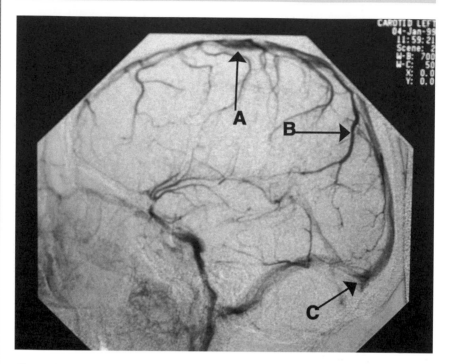

Question 3

1. What is this investigation?
2. Name structure A.
3. Name structure B.
4. Name structure C.
5. What is the volume of contrast and the rate of infusion normally used for this study?

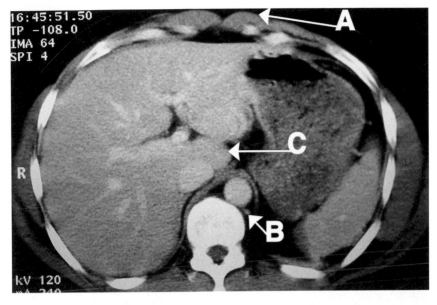

Question 4

1. Name structure A.
2. Name structure B.
3. Which liver segment does C refer to?
4. What does TP indicate?
5. What does a pitch of 1.5 refer to?

Exam I

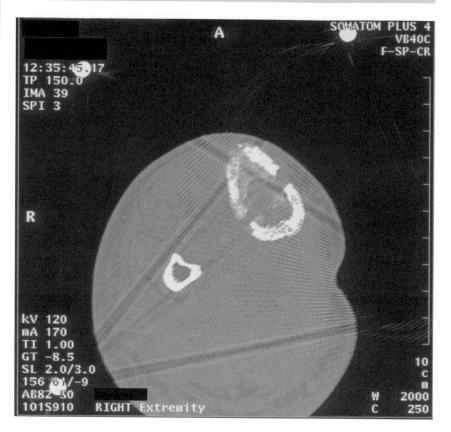

Question 5

1. What is this investigation?
2. What causes the array of lines across the image?
3. What is the source of the 'lines'?
4. In CT, what is meant by beam–hardening artefact and where does it typically occur?
5. How is beam hardening effectively dealt with?

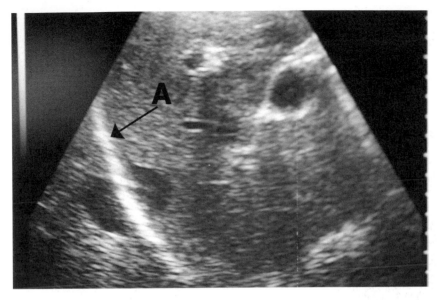

Question 6

1. What artefact is demonstrated?
2. Why does it occur?
3. Name structure A.
4. What is the most likely type of probe used for this investigation?
5. What is the patient preparation for imaging the gall bladder and why?

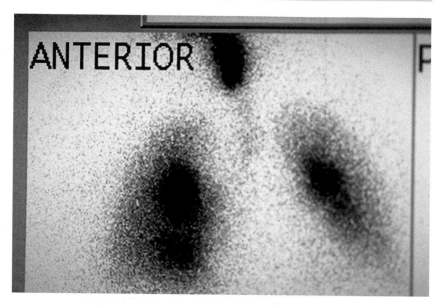

Question 7

1. What investigation is this and why?
2. Name three radiopharmaceuticals that may be used for this part of the study.
3. Name one contraindication when performing this investigation.
4. What views should be routinely performed?
5. What is the position of the gamma camera in this patient?

Exam I

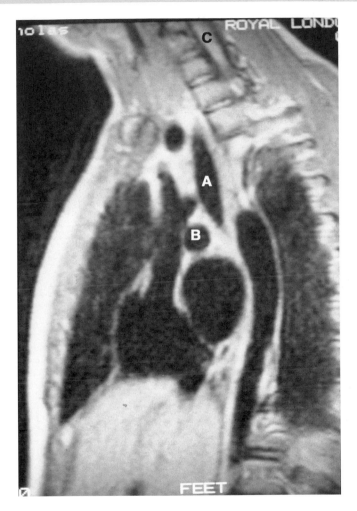

Question 8

1. Name structure A.
2. Name structure B.
3. Name structure C.
4. How is cardiac motion artefact minimized during this investigation?
5. In which direction is motion artefact usually visible?

Exam I

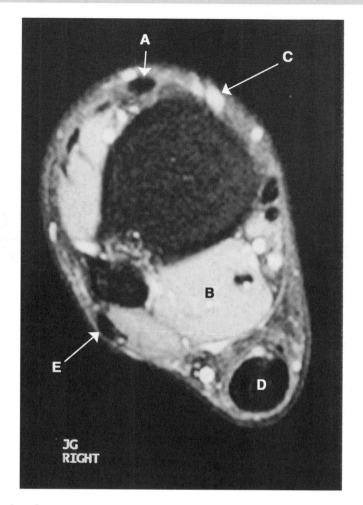

JG
RIGHT

Question 9

1. Name structure A.
2. Name structure B.
3. Name structure C.
4. Name structure D.
5. Name structure E.

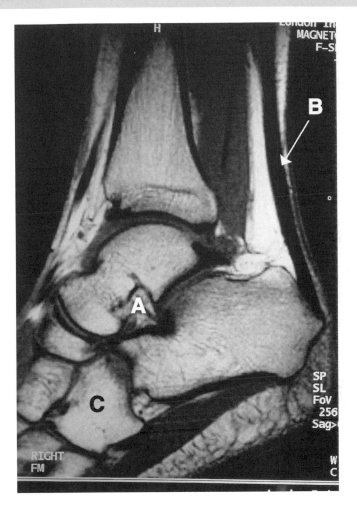

Question 10

1. Name structure A.
2. Name structure B.
3. Name structure C.
4. What is the best imaging plane to demonstrate the deltoid ligament?
5. Do tissues with a short T1 appear as high signal or low signal on a T1 W image?

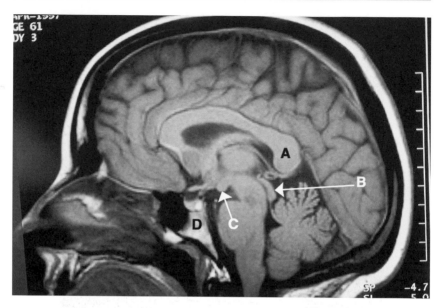

Question 11

1. Name structure A.
2. Name structure B.
3. Name structure C.
4. Explain whether or not gadolinium has been given.
5. Name structure D. Why does it return a high signal?

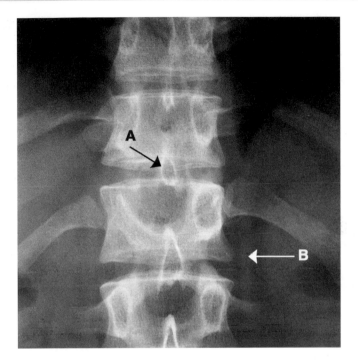

Question 12

1. What is the normal variant demonstrated?
2. Name structure A.
3. Name structure B.
4. What is the centering point for an AP lumbar spine X-ray?
5. What makes structure B visible?

Exam I

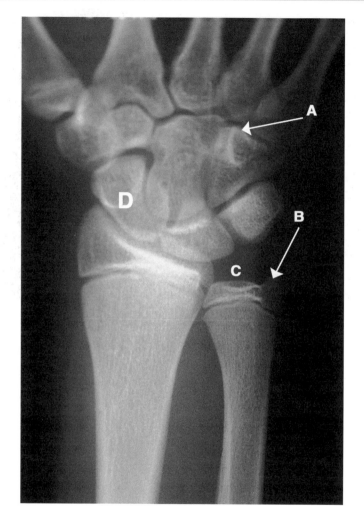

Question 13

1. Name structure A.
2. Name structure B.
3. Which structure lies in the space denoted by C?
4. Which carpal bone ossifies first and which ossifies last?
5. Name structure D, and what is interesting about its blood supply?

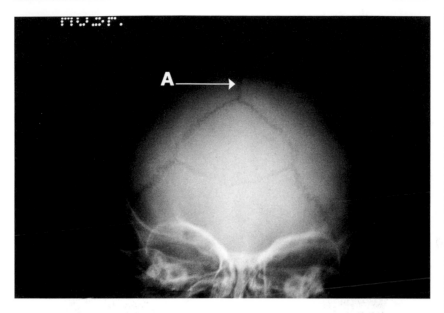

Question 14

1. What is the normal variant shown?
2. In what bone does it lie?
3. Name structure A.
4. What is the maximal suture width in subjects of the following ages:
   - (i)   birth?
   - (ii)   2 years of age?
   - (iii)   3 years of age?
5. In which bones do the following sutures lie:
   - (i)   metopic suture?
   - (ii)   mendosal suture?

Exam 1

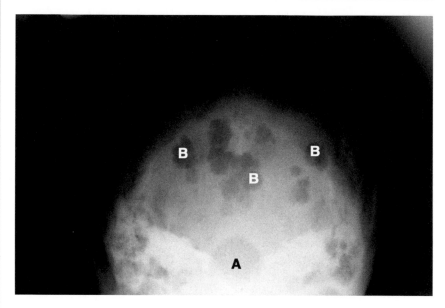

Question 15

1. What view is this?
2. Name structure A.
3. What cranial nerve passes through A and in which direction does it travel?
4. Name structure B.
5. What is the function of structure B?

Exam 1

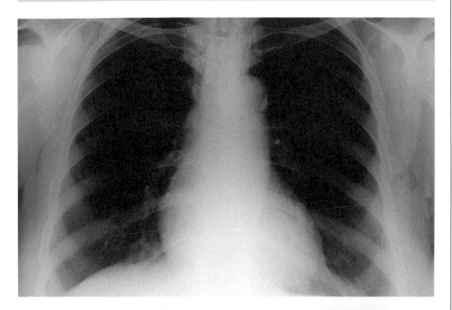

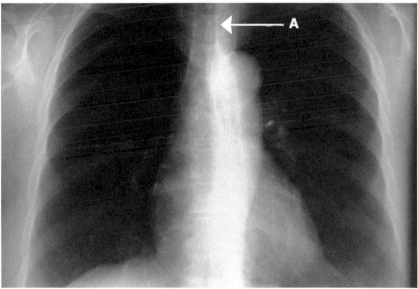

Question 16

1. What is the difference between these two films?
2. How can one differentiate between the two?
3. Give a typical kV for each of these two studies.
4. On the lower film name structure A.
5. What causes A?

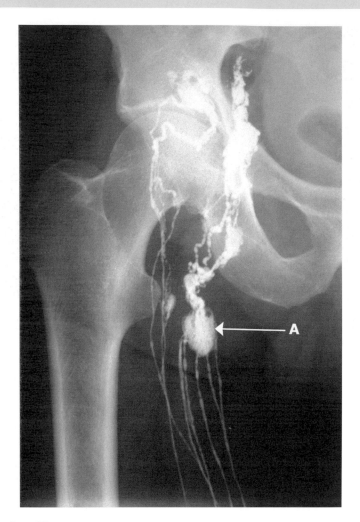

Question 17

1. What is the usual site of injection of contrast for this study?
2. Name two contrast agents suitable for this investigation.
3. How do these two agents differ in their pattern of opacification?
4. In unilateral cannulation, which side is usually cannulated and why?
5. Name structure A.

Exam 1

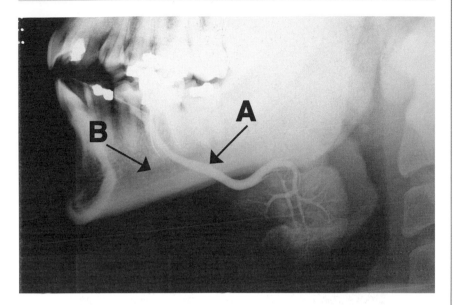

Question 18

1. What is this investigation?
2. Where is the tip of the cannula sited?
3. Name structure A.
4. What structures run in B?
5. Which control films are done and why?

Exam 1

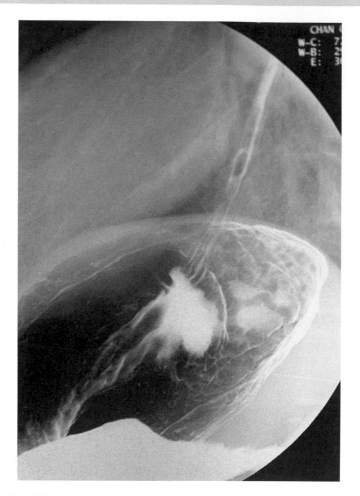

Question 19

1. In what position is the patient?
2. Give two contraindications to using Buscopan.
3. What alternative medication may be used if Buscopan is contraindicated?
4. What other patient position may be used to visualise this part of the stomach?
5. What is the recommended volume of gas used for this investigation?

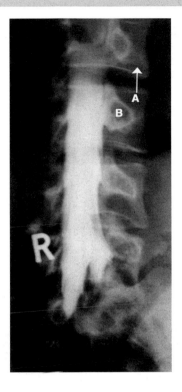

Question 20

1. Name structure A.
2. Name structure B.
3. Give two complications of this procedure.
4. Describe the appearance of contrast injected into the following dural spaces:
   (i) subdural space.
   (ii) extradural space.
5. What advice should be given to a patient after a myelogram?

Answers – Exam 1

Question I

1. This is a selective superior mesenteric artery arteriogram.
2. Catheters: Sidewinder, Simmons, femorovisceral.
3. 42 ml of contrast at 7 ml per second is appropriate.
4. A = ripple effect in the arteries. This occurs due to rapid injections of contrast.
5. Contrast is identified in the renal pelvis, which indicates that this is not the first injection of contrast.

Question 2

1. This is a right-sided ascending venogram.
2. A = right long saphenous vein.
3. B = venous valve in the right superficial femoral vein.
4. Low osmolar contrast medium – 240–300 mg I/ml should be used.
5. Alternative investigations: Doppler ultrasound scan/magnetic resonance venography.

Question 3

1. This is the venous phase of a cerebral angiogram (DSA).
2. A = superior sagittal sinus.
3. B = vein of Trollard.
4. C = torcula herophili.
5. 6 ml of contrast is infused at 1.5 ml per second.

Question 4

1. A = left rectus abdominis muscle.
2. B = hemiazygous vein.
3. C = caudate lobe (segment I).
4. TP = table position.
5. Pitch of 1.5 = collimation of one slice multiplied by a factor of 1.5.

Question 5

1. This is an axial CT through the right lower leg viewed on bony windows.
2. The array of lines is secondary to star artefact from metallic objects.
3. The source of the artefact is the frame of the external fixator which is just visible in cross-section at the extremities of the image.
4. Beam hardening: progressive removal of low kV components of the CT beam as it traverses tissue. This gives rise to an artefactual increase in the effective energy of the beam resulting in a decrease in the CT number of the tissue. Beam hardening is typically seen in the posterior fossa due to the petrous ridges.
5. Using a beam-hardening algorithm reduces beam-hardening artefact.

Question 6

1. The artefact demonstrated is a mirror image artefact.
2. Mirror image artefact occurs in a region that has strong reflectors, such as the diaphragm. The echoes lying to one side of this strong reflector are interpreted as arising on both sides of it and an image of the liver is produced lying within the lung.
3. A = diaphragm.
4. Transducer: curvilinear 3.5 MHz.
5. Patient preparation: the patient should be fasted in order to distend the gallbladder prior to scanning.

Question 7

1. This is a ventilation perfusion radionuclide scan. This particular image demonstrates the ventilation aspect of the study, identified by the presence of radionuclide tracer within the oropharynx and trachea.
2. Radiopharmaceuticals:
    (i) ^{81m}krypton.
    (ii) ^{99m}Tc-DPTA.
    (iii) ^{133}Xe.
3. Contraindications:
    (i)   right-to-left shunt.
    (ii) severe pulmonary hypertension.
4. Routine views: anterior/posterior/RPO/LPO.
5. For an anterior image, the gamma camera is placed in front of the patient. For a posterior image, the gamma camera is placed behind the patient.

Question 8

1. A = trachea.
2. B = right pulmonary artery.
3. C = cervical spinal cord.
4. Cardiac motion artefact is minimized by using cardiac gating. Each pulse sequence is triggered by an 'R' wave, where TR = the R–R interval.
5. Motion artefact is usually visible in the phase-encoding direction.

Question 9

1. A = tendon of tibialis anterior.
2. B = flexor hallucis longus muscle.
3. C = long saphenous vein.
4. D = tendoachilles.
5. E = tendon of peroneus longus.

Question 10

1. A = sinus tarsi.
2. B = tendocalcaneus (aka Achilles tendon).
3. C = cuboid.
4. The deltoid ligament is best imaged in a coronal plane.
5. Structures with a short T1 appear as high signal on T1 W imaging.

Question 11

1. A = splenium of the corpus callosum.
2. B = quadrigeminal plate.
3. C = mamillary body.
4. Gadolinium has not been given. Following gadolinium, normal mucosa would return a high signal on a T1 sequence.
5. D = clivus: it returns a high signal as it contains marrow fat.

Question 12

1. There is an absent right pedicle of T12.
2. A = spinous process of T11.
3. B = crus of the left diaphragm.
4. Centering point = midline at the lower costal margin.
5. The crus is visible due to the silhouette sign, i.e. fat lies adjacent to the crus, making it visible.

Question 13

1. A = hook of hamate.
2. B = ulnar styloid process.
3. The triangular fibrocartilage complex lies in the space denoted by C.
4. The capitate ossifies first, the pisiform ossifies last.
5. D = scaphoid bone. The blood supply arises from its distal pole and the scaphoid is prone to avascular necrosis when fractured.

Question 14

1. The normal variant demonstrated is an inca bone.
2. The inca bone lies within the occipital bone.
3. A = sagittal suture.
4. Maximum suture width:
    (i) birth = 10 mm.
    (ii) 2 years = 3 mm.
    (iii) 3 years = 2 mm.
5. (i) The metopic sutures lies within the frontal bone.
    (ii) The mendosal suture lies within the occipital bone.

Question 15

1. This is a Towne's view.
2. A = foramen magnum.
3. The spinal part of the accessory cranial nerve passes through the foramen magnum in a cranial direction.
4. B = arachnoid granulations.
5. The function of the arachnoid granulations is CSF resorption.

Question 16

1. The upper film has been taken at low kV whilst the lower film has been taken at high kV.
2. The ribs are better visualised on the upper film whilst the soft tissues are under penetrated. On the lower film, however, the ribs are poorly visualised and there has been better penetration of the soft tissues allowing clearer identification of lung markings.
3. Low kV, 65 kV; high kV, 120 kV.
4. A = posterior junctional line.
5. The posterior junctional line is formed as a result of both lungs meeting in the midline posteriorly.

Question 17

1. This is a lymphangiogram. Contrast medium is usually injected into the first or second web spaces of the right foot.
2. Contrast agents:
   Lipiodol
   Omnipaque
3. Lipiodol is oily – it opacifies both lymphatic vessels and lymph nodes. Omnipaque is water soluble – it opacifies the lymphatic vessels only.
4. Cannulation is usually performed in the right leg, due to the greater natural left to right lymphatic crossover that exists in the body. Hence, there is greater flow in the right lymphatic system.
5. A = Deep Inguinal node.

Question 18

1. This is a submandibular sialogram.
2. The tip of the cannula is sited beside the frenulum in the floor of the mouth.
3. A = Wharton's duct.
4. The inferior alveolar nerve and artery run in B (inferior alveolar canal).
5. Control films:
      (i)   lateral view with tongue depressed.
      (ii) lateral oblique.
      (iii) occlusal films.
These are performed to identify calculi on preliminary films.

Question 19

1. The patient is in a left lateral position.
2. Contraindications to Buscopan: glaucoma and cardiac arrhythmias.
3. Glucagon may be administered in the event of a contraindication to Buscopan.
4. To visualise the gastric fundus, further views may be taken with the patient erect.
5. 200–400 ml of gas is recommended.

Question 20

1. A = right transverse process of L2.
2. B = right pedicle of L3.
3. Complications:
      (i)   hypotension.
      (ii) headaches.
      (iii) neural toxicity.
      (iv) back pain.
      (v)   haemorrhage.
4.   (i)   Subdural space – the contrast remains as a small 'pool' around the needle tip.
     (ii) Extradural space – the contrast outlines the nerve roots beyond the exit foramina.
5. Post-myelogram, the patient should be advised to maintain a high fluid intake and remain ambulant.

Exam 2

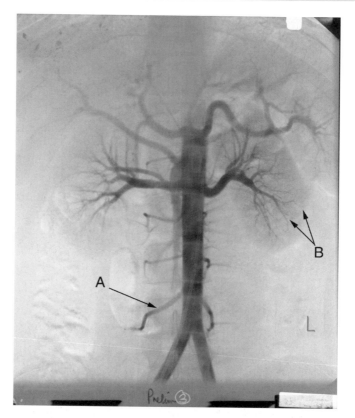

Question 1

1. What is this investigation?
2. What types of catheter are normally used?
3. Name structure A.
4. Name structure B.
5. What percentage of the population have accessory renal arteries?

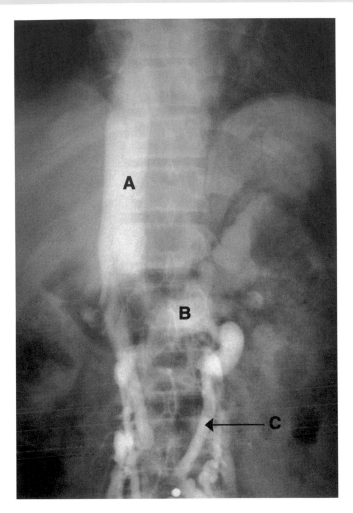

Question 2

1. What is this investigation?
2. What would be a suitable injection site, volume and rate of contrast administration for this study?
3. Name structure A.
4. Name structure B.
5. Name structure C.

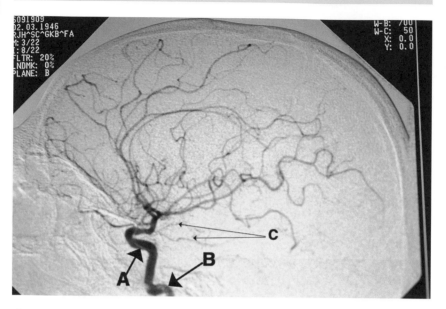

Question 3

1. What is this investigation?
2. Name structure A.
3. Name structure B.
4. Name structure C.
5. Name two local complications of femoral artery puncture.

Exam 2

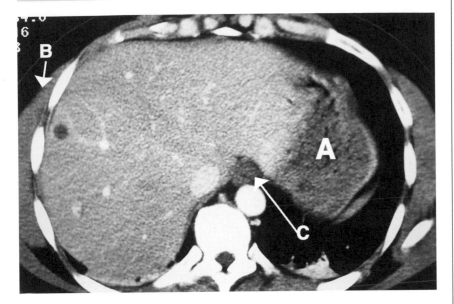

Question 4

1. Name structure A.
2. Has the patient received oral contrast?
3. Name structure B.
4. Name the three phases of CT imaging of the liver and give the approximate times when these phases are performed.
5. Name structure C.

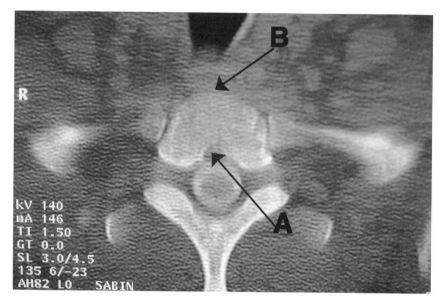

Question 5

1. What is this investigation?
2. In which space does the contrast lie?
3. Describe two other methods of assessing nerve roots.
4. What is the cause of the indentation at A?
5. Which ligament is attached to B?

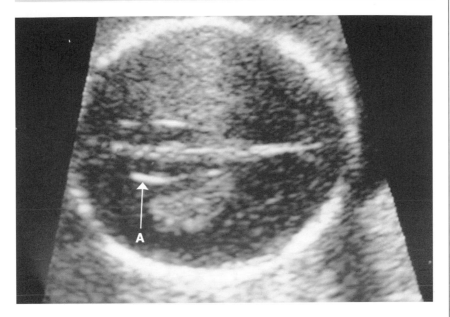

Question 6

1. What is this investigation?
2. Name structure A.
3. Name two measurements performed on this image.
4. At what level is the biparietal diameter measured (BPD)?
5. At what age do the anterior and posterior fontanelles close?

Exam 2

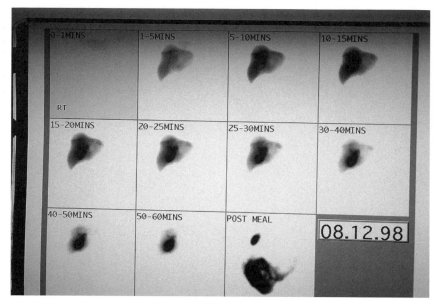

Question 7

1. What is this investigation?
2. Give the typical administered dose and radioisotope used.
3. Which cells routinely take up the radiopharmaceutical?
4. What are the indications for this scan?
5. What is the route of administration for this radiopharmaceutical?

Exam 2

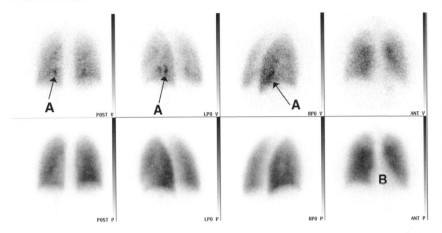

Question 8

1. What is the cause for appearance A?
2. What does B represent?
3. What is the most likely ventilation agent used here?
4. What is the half-life of ^{81m}krypton gas?
5. Which perfusion agent is routinely used?

Exam 2

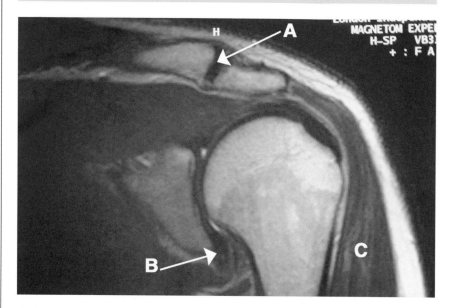

Question 9

1. What is this investigation?
2. Name structure A.
3. Name structure B.
4. Name structure C. Is it part of the rotator cuff complex?
5. Name the components of the rotator cuff complex.

Exam 2

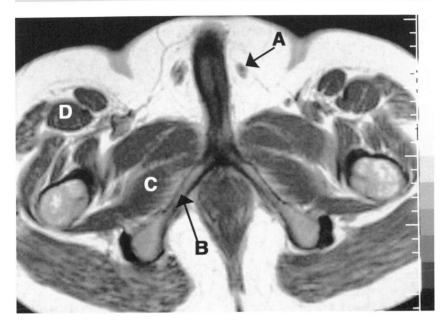

Question 10

1. Name structure A.
2. Name structure B.
3. Name structure C.
4. Where does structure D originate from?
5. The zonal anatomy of the prostate gland is best seen on which MRI sequence?

Exam 2

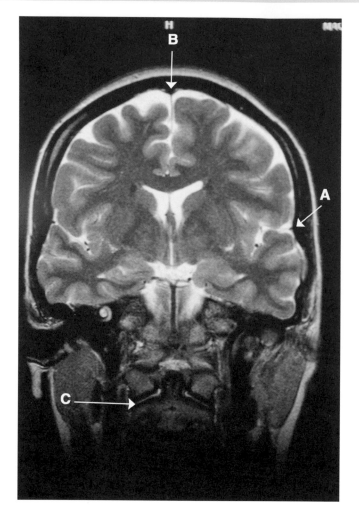

Question 11

1. What sequence has been performed?
2. Name structure A.
3. Name structure B. Why is it of low signal?
4. Name structure C.
5. Would this film appear in a standard MRI study of the brain?

Exam 2

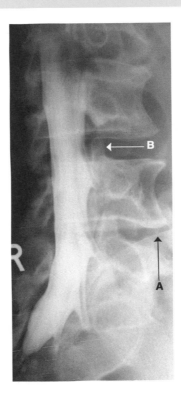

Question 12

1. What view has been taken?
2. If this view is a posterior projection, which neural foramina would be best demonstrated?
3. Name structure A.
4. Name structure B.
5. Name two other methods of imaging spinal nerve roots.

Exam 2

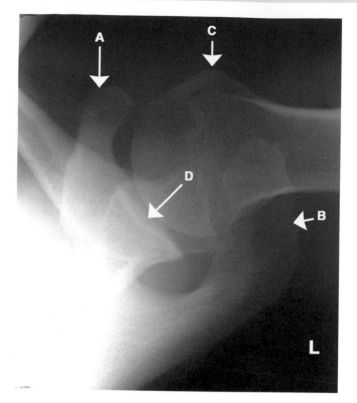

Question 13

1. What view is demonstrated?
2. Name structure A.
3. Name structure B.
4. Name structure C.
5. Name structure D.

Exam 2

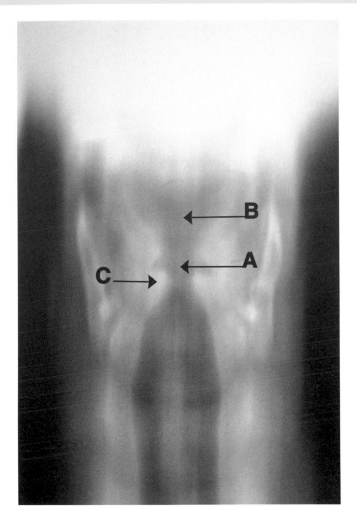

Question 14

1. What is this investigation?
2. Name structure A.
3. Name structure B.
4. Name structure C.
5. What other imaging modality is commonly used to assess this area?

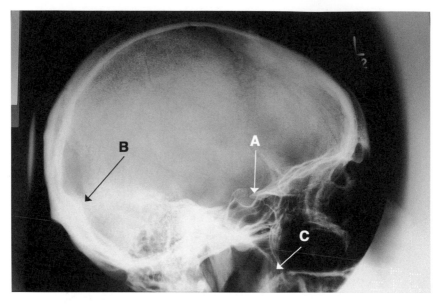

Question 15

1. Name structure A.
2. Name structure B.
3. Name structure C.
4. Which vessels meet at point B and what do they form?
5. Name five normal structures that may calcify in the brain.

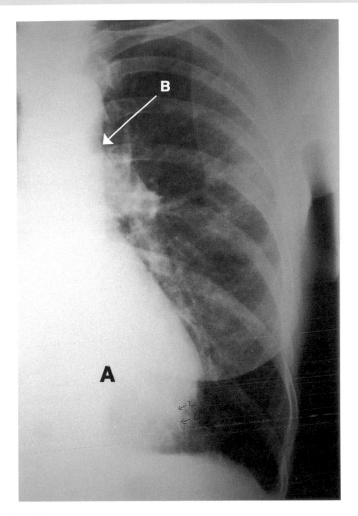

Question 16

1. Which heart chamber does A represent?
2. Name structure B.
3. Name four structures normally found in structure B.
4. Which hilum is normally higher?
5. Is the radiographic technique adequate for this PA film?

Exam 2

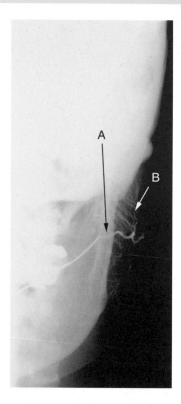

Question 17

1. What is this investigation?
2. Where is contrast injected?
3. Name structure A.
4. Name structure B.
5. Name the main contraindication to this procedure.

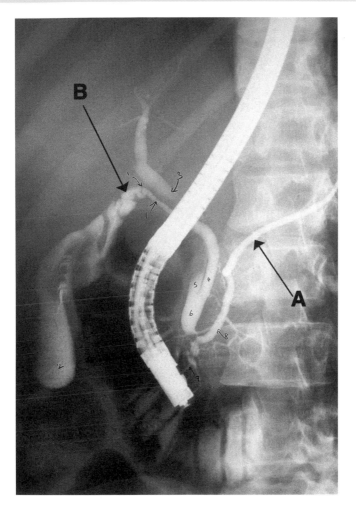

Question 18

1. What is this investigation?
2. Give two indications for this test.
3. Give two contraindications.
4. Name structure A.
5. Name structure B.

Exam 2

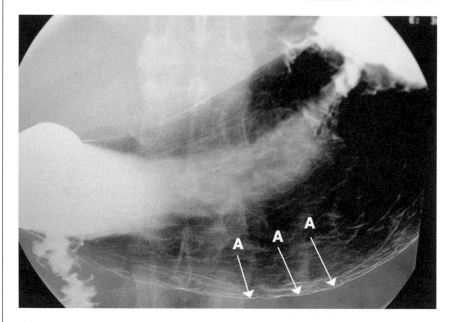

Question 19

1. What is this investigation?
2. What position is the patient in?
3. Name structure A.
4. What concentration of barium is commonly used for this investigation?
5. What is the approximate duration of action of Buscopan?

Exam 2

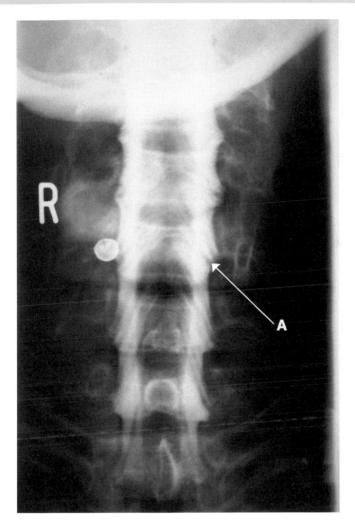

Question 20

1. Name structure A.
2. (i) Where does the C3 nerve root emerge?
   (ii) Where does the T1 nerve root emerge?
3. Name two methods by which contrast may be introduced in this area.
4. What is the patient position for a lateral cervical puncture?
5. Name two contraindications to lateral cervical puncture.

Question 1

1. This is a flush aortogram.
2. Catheters used: straight/pigtail catheters.
3. A = lowest right lumbar artery.
4. B = arcuate vessels left kidney.
5. 25% of the population has accessory renal arteries.

Question 2

1. This is an inferior venocavogram.
2. 40 ml of contrast is injected via the femoral vein at 2 ml per second.
3. A = Inferior vena cava.
4. B = Left renal vein.
5. C = Left ascending lumbar vein.

Question 3

1. This is a selective internal carotid arteriogram.
2. A = cavernous portion of internal carotid artery.
3. B = petrous portion of internal carotid artery.
4. C = anterior choroidal artery.
5. Local complications:
   (i) haematoma.
   (ii) false aneurysms.
   (iii) damage to adjacent structures.
   (iv) infection.

Question 4

1. A = stomach.
2. The patient has not been given any oral contrast.
3. B = right serratus anterior.
4. Three phases:
   (i) precontrast.
   (ii) arterial phase – about 30 seconds.
   (iii) portal venous phase – about 60 seconds.
5. C = oesophagus.

Question 5

1. This is a CT myelogram.
2. Contrast is injected into the subarachnoid space.
3. Alternatively, nerve roots may be assessed by myelography and MRI.
4. A = indentation caused by the basivertebral vein.
5. The anterior longitudinal ligament is attached at B.

Question 6

1. This is an ultrasound scan of the foetal head.
2. A = lateral wall of cavum septum pellucidum.
3. Measurements performed on the foetal head:
    (i)   biparietal diameter.
    (ii) total head circumference.
    (iii) size of cerebellum/ventricular ratio.
4. The BPD is measured at the level of the thalamus/septum pellucidum.
5. The posterior fontanelle closes at 6 months of age whilst the anterior fontanelle closes at 18 months of age.

Question 7

1. This is a dynamic radionuclide hepatobiliary scan (cholescintigraphy).
2. The typical administered dose is 75 MBq (150 MBq maximum). The agent most commonly used is ^{99m}Tc-HIDA.
3. The radiolabelled derivatives of HIDA are rapidly cleared from the circulation by hepatocytes and secreted into bile in a similar way to bilirubin.
4. (i)   Suspected acute cholecystitis.
    (ii) Diagnosis and location of biliary obstruction after a negative ultrasound.
    (iii) Neonatal jaundice (?atresia).
    (iv) Suspected bile leaks.
5. The patient lies supine with the camera anterior and the liver at the top of the field of view. The radiopharmaceutical is injected intravenously.

Question 8

1. A represents clumping of aerosol particles in the ventilation phase of scanning.
2. B is a relatively photon-deficient area due to the heart.
3. The most likely agent used here is ^{99m}DPTA aerosol, as there has been clumping of aerosol particles within the lung.
4. Half-life of ^{81m}krypton gas = 13 seconds.
5. Perfusion agent: ^{99m}Tc-macro aggregates of albumin.

Question 9

1. This is a coronal T1W MRI of the shoulder.
2. A = left acromioclavicular joint.
3. B = left inferior glenoid labrum.
4. C = left deltoid muscle. This is not part of the rotator cuff complex.
5. Rotator cuff complex: supraspinatus, infraspinatus, teres minor and subscapularis muscles.

Question 10

1. A = left spermatic cord.
2. B = right inferior pubic ramus.
3. C = right obturator externus muscle.
4. D = rectus femoris muscle. This arises from the anterior inferior iliac spine.
5. The zonal anatomy of the prostate is best seen on T2 W images.

Question 11

1. This is a coronal T2 W MRI of the brain.
2. A = left sylvian fissure.
3. B = superior sagittal sinus. This is of low signal secondary to a flow void.
4. C = right lateral atlantoaxial joint.
5. This is not a standard MRI sequence of the brain. Axial and sagittal images are routine images in this study.

Question 12

1. This is an oblique view of the lumbar spine.
2. A right posterior oblique of the lumbar spine would demonstrate the left intervertebral foramina.
3. A = iliac crest.
4. B = superior articular facet of L4.
5. Spinal nerve roots may also be imaged using CT myelography and MRI.

Question 13

1. This is an axial view of the left shoulder.
2. A = left coracoid process.
3. B = left acromion process.
4. C = lesser tuberosity of the left humerus.
5. D = left glenoid fossa.

Question 14

1. This is a coronal laryngeal tomogram.
2. A = ventricle.
3. B = vestibule.
4. C = true cords.
5. CT is now commonly used to image this area.

Question 15

1. A = anterior clinoid process.
2. B = internal occipital protuberance.
3. C = pterygoid plates.
4. The superior sagittal sinus and the straight sinus meet at point B. They form the right and left transverse sinuses.
5. Structures that normally calcify in the brain:
   - (i) carotid artery.
   - (ii) habenular commissure.
   - (iii) petroclinoid ligament.
   - (iv) interclinoid ligament.
   - (v) pineal gland.
   - (vi) falx cerebri.
   - (vii) tentorium cerebelli.
   - (viii) basal ganglia.
   - (ix) choroid plexus.

Question 16

1. A = right ventricle.
2. B = aortopulmonary window.
3. Four structures normally found in the aortopulmonary window are:
   - (i) lymph nodes.
   - (ii) ligamentum arteriosum.
   - (iii) left recurrent laryngeal nerve (branch of the vagus nerve).
   - (iv) mediastinal fat.

   The thymus may be found here in adolescents.
4. The left hilum is normally higher than the right.
5. There has been a suboptimal technique here as the medial border of the scapula is still projected over the left lateral chest wall.

Question 17

1. This is a left parotid sialogram.
2. Contrast is injected into the orifice of Stensen's duct opposite the 2nd upper molar tooth.
3. A = Stensen's duct.
4. B = secondary ductules.
5. Contraindication: acute infection/inflammation.

Question 18

1. This is an ERCP.
2. Indications:
    (i) extrahepatic biliary obstruction.
    (ii) postcholecystectomy syndrome.
    (iii) pancreatic disease.
    (iv) diffuse biliary disease.
3. Contraindications:
    (i) acute pancreatitis.
    (ii) previous gastric surgery.
    (iii) oesophageal obstruction.
    (iv) HIV/hepatitis B.
    (v) pancreatic pseudocyst.
    (vi) severe cardiorespiratory disease.
4. A = pancreatic duct.
5. B = neck of gall bladder.

Question 19

1. This is a double-contrast barium meal examination.
2. The patient is supine.
3. A = greater curvature of the stomach.
4. Concentration of barium: EZHD-250% w/v.
5. Buscopan has a duration of action of 15 minutes.

Question 20

1. A = left C5 nerve root.
2. (i) The C3 nerve root emerges between C2 and C3.
    (ii) The T1 nerve root emerges between T1 and T2.
3. Contrast may be introduced via a lateral cervical puncture or by 'run-up' from a lumbar puncture.
4. The patient is in a prone position for a lateral cervical puncture.
5. Contraindications:
    (i) suspected upper cervical mass lesion.
    (ii) suspected lumbar spinal dysraphism.
    (iii) loss of the C1–2 intervertebral space secondary to spinal deformity.

Exam 3

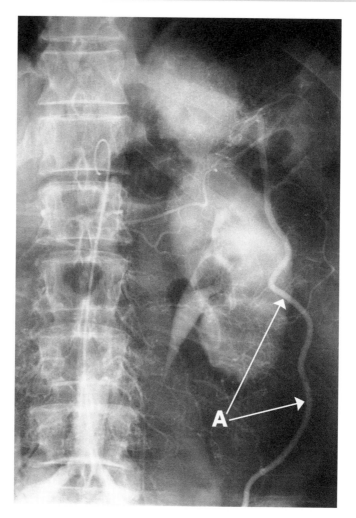

Question 1

1. Name structure A.
2. Where does A normally arise from?
3. For this investigation, what is the puncture site?
4. What are the normal anatomical relations of the puncture vessel in the groin?
5. What is the minimal rate of bleeding for a selective angiogram to be positive?

Exam 3

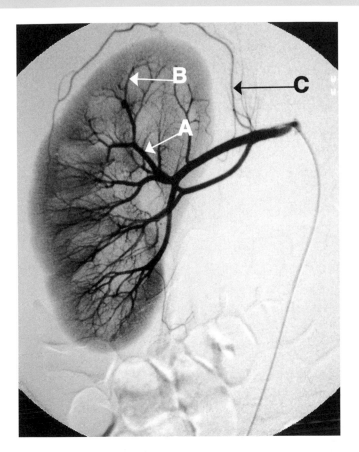

Question 2

1. What is this investigation?
2. What type of catheters can be used?
3. Name structures A and B.
4. Name structure C.
5. Summarize the blood supply to the adrenal gland.

Exam 3

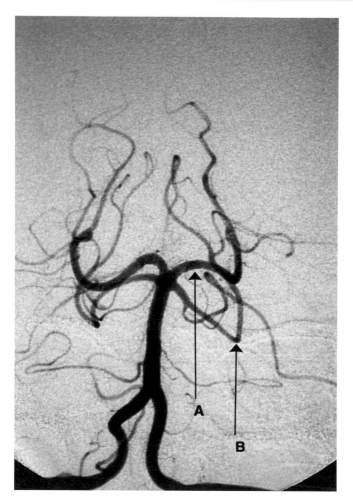

Question 3

1. What investigation is this and where is the catheter tip most likely to be?
2. Name a possible catheter, volume of contrast and rate of contrast infusion that may be used for this investigation.
3. Which cistern is vessel A lying in?
4. Name structure B.
5. Name a specific operative complication unique to this study.

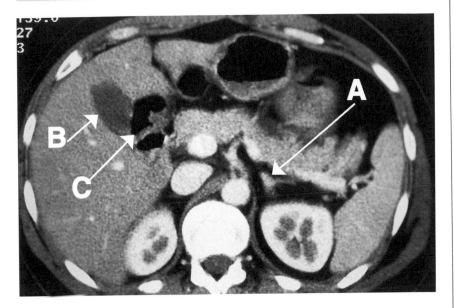

Question 4

1. Name structure A.
2. What are the normal dimensions of structure A?
3. Name structure B.
4. Name structure C.
5. At what phase of renal scanning has this image been taken and what is the appropriate delay prior to imaging?

Exam 3

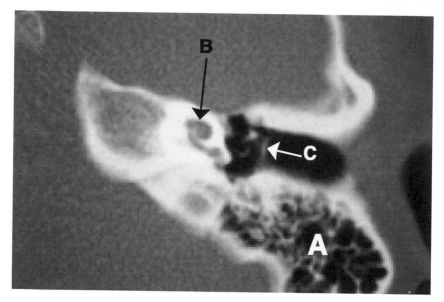

Question 5

1. Name structure A.
2. Name structure B.
3. Within which bone does the inner ear lie?
4. Name structure C.
5. Give an appropriate slice thickness and pitch for this investigation.

Exam 3

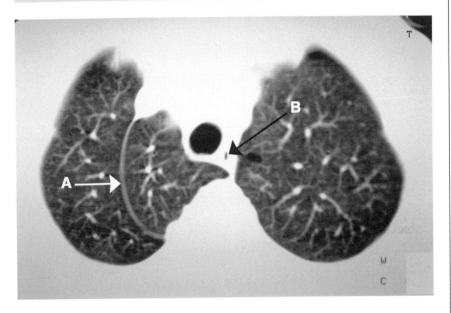

Question 6

1. Name structure A.
2. In what percentage of the population does structure A occur?
3. How many layers of pleura is structure A formed from?
4. Name structure B.
5. What do the letters W and C in the bottom right-hand corner of the image refer to? Give an appropriate figure for each of these letters.

Exam 3

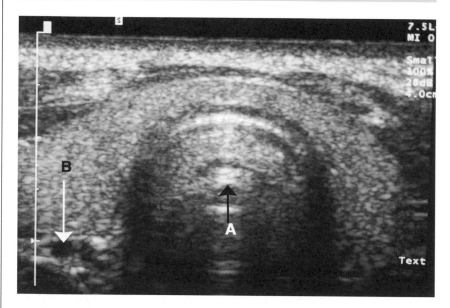

Question 7

1. What is this investigation?
2. What frequency transducer is commonly used?
3. What causes the echogenic crescent A?
4. What does B represent?
5. What position should the patient be in for this scan?

Exam 3

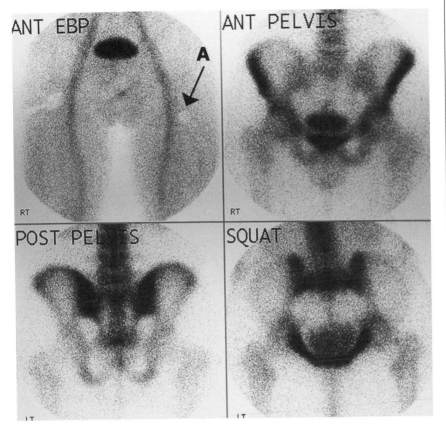

Question 8

1. From what investigation are these images taken?
2. What does EBP indicate?
3. Suggest a cause for the photon-deficient area marked A.
4. What is the usual administered dose of radionuclide for this study?
5. What are the different phases for this investigation and at what times are they imaged?

Exam 3

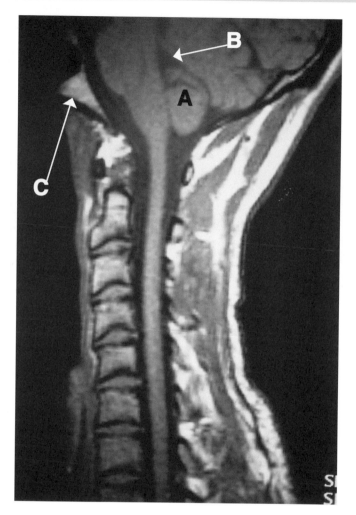

Question 9

1. What is this investigation?
2. Name structure A.
3. Name structure B.
4. Name structure C.
5. Why is structure C of high signal?

Exam 3

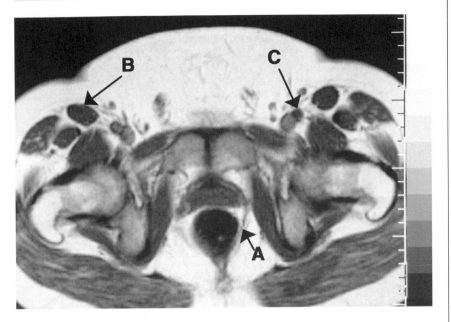

Question 10

1. Name structure A.
2. Name structure B.
3. Name structure C.
4. How is the total time of an MR sequence calculated?
5. Give approximate values for TF and TR for a T1-weighted MRI.

Exam 3

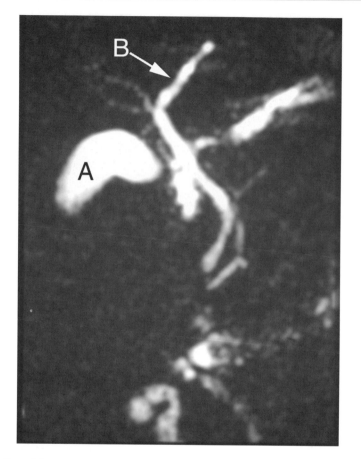

Question 11

1. What is this investigation?
2. What sequence is used?
3. Is gadolinium required?
4. Name structure A.
5. Name structure B.

Exam 3

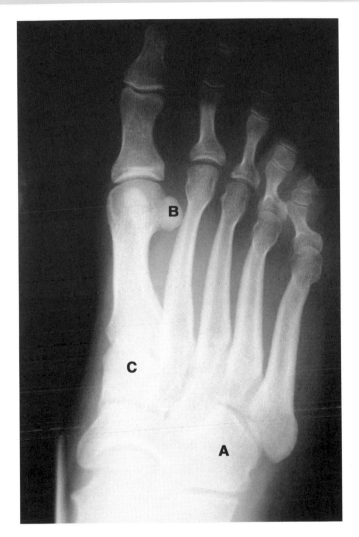

Question 12

1. Name structure A.
2. Name structure B.
3. In what structure does B normally lie?
4. What is the centering point for this view?
5. Name structure C.

Exam 3

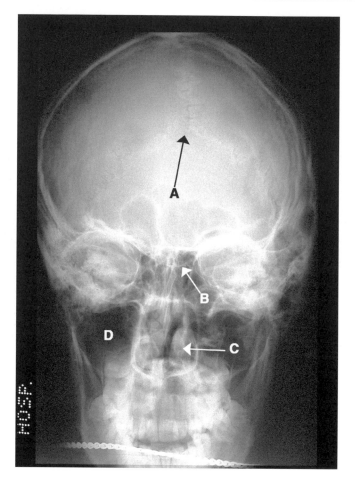

Question 13

1. What view is demonstrated and how is this assessed?
2. Name structure A.
3. Name structure B.
4. Name structure C.
5. Which space is related to the posterior aspect of structure D?

Exam 3

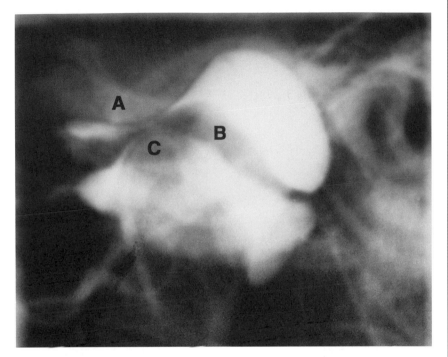

Question 14

1. Name structure A.
2. Name structure B.
3. Name structure C.
4. Is the mouth open or closed and how do you know?
5. What muscle attaches to B?

Exam 3

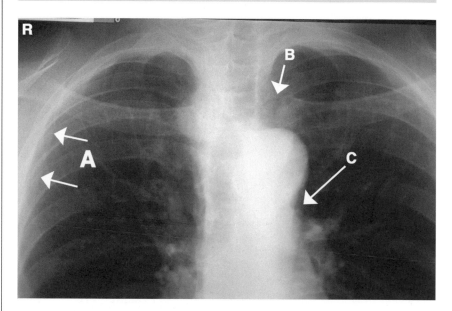

Question 15

1. Comment on the technical quality of this film.
2. Name structure A.
3. What type of joint is B?
4. What structure produces lines C?
5. What is a typical kV for this chest X-ray?

Exam 3

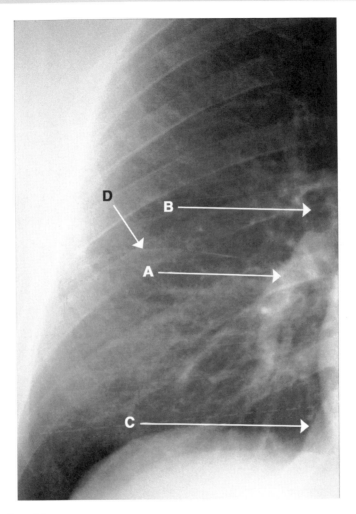

Question 16

1. Name structure A.
2. What is the normal size of structure A?
3. (i) Name point B.
   (ii) Which vessels form the angle at point B?
   (iii) What is the normal angle at point B?
4. Name structure C.
5. Name structure D.

Exam 3

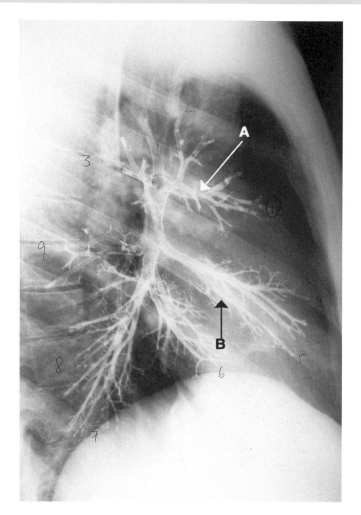

Question 17

1. Which view has been performed?
2. Name two contraindications to this study.
3. Name two complications related to this investigation.
4. Name structure A.
5. Name structure B.

Exam 3

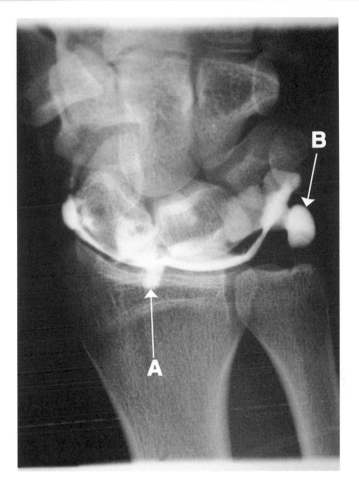

Question 18

1. What is this study?
2. How much contrast is injected and where is it introduced?
3. Name structure A.
4. Name structure B.
5. What is the normal intercarpal joint distance?

Exam 3

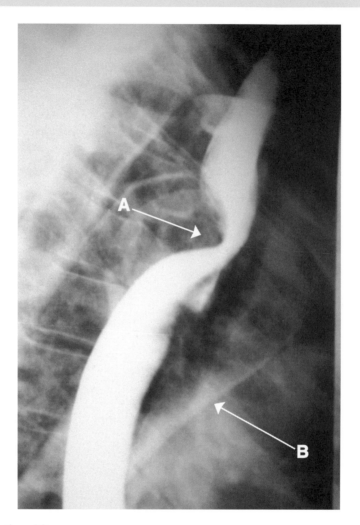

Question 19

1. What is this study? Give two indications for this test to be performed.
2. What concentration of barium is routinely used?
3. Give two contraindications to the initial use of barium for this investigation.
4. What causes the indentation A?
5. Name structure B.

Exam 3

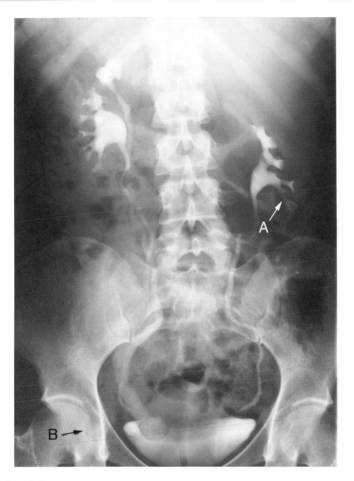

Question 20

1. What is the normal variant demonstrated?
2. In approximately what percentage of the population does this variant occur?
3. Name structure A.
4. Name structure B.
5. Name three contraindications to abdominal compression in an IVU.

Question 1

1. A = Wandering (marginal) artery of Drummond.
2. The marginal artery usually arises from the left colic artery (a branch of the IMA).
3. The puncture site is the femoral artery.
4. The relations of the femoral artery in the groin are:
   (i)   medial - femoral vein.
   (ii) lateral - femoral nerve.
5. A rate of GI bleeding as low as 0.5 ml per minute can be detected by selective angiography.

Question 2

1. This is a selective renal angiogram (DSA).
2. Catheters: Femororenal/Simmonds.
3. A = lobar artery, B = arcuate artery.
4. C = inferior adrenal artery arising from the renal artery.
5. Blood supply to the adrenal gland:
   (i)   superior adrenal artery – branch of the inferior phrenic artery.
   (ii) middle adrenal artery – branch of the aorta.
   (iii) inferior adrenal artery – branch of the renal artery.

Question 3

1. This is a vertebral digital subtraction angiogram. The catheter tip is most likely to lie in the left vertebral artery.
2. Catheter: Headhunter/Newton/Mani.
   Volume of contrast administered is 6 ml.
   Rate of administration: contrast is usually given via hand injection.
3. A = posterior cerebral artery which is found in the ambient cistern.
4. B = left superior cerebellar artery.
5. Cortical blindness is a specific complication unique to this study.

Question 4

1. A = body of the left adrenal gland.
2. Normal dimensions:
   (i)   body – 1 cm.
   (ii) limb thickness – 4 mm.
   (iii) height – 4 cm.
3. B = gall bladder.
4. C = second part of duodenum.
5. This image has been taken in the corticomedullary phase. A delay of approximately 30 seconds would be appropriate for this image.

Question 5

1. A = mastoid air cells.
2. B = cochlea.
3. The cochlea lies within the petrous part of the temporal bone.
4. C = tympanic membrane.
5. For CT of the petrous temporal bone: slice = 2–3 mm, pitch = 1–1.5 mm.

Question 6

1. A = azygous fissure.
2. An azygous fissure is seen in 0.4% of chest X-rays and is found in 1% of postmortem examinations.
3. The azygous fissure consists of four layers of pleura.
4. B = oesophagus.
5. W = window width, C = centre (aka window level). W = 1600, C = –600.

Question 7

1. This is a thyroid ultrasound scan.
2. A 7.5 MHz linear transducer is routinely used.
3. A = air in the trachea.
4. B = blood vessels in the right lobe of the thyroid.
5. Position: supine, neck extended.

Question 8

1. ^{99m}Tc-MDP bone scan. The images are of the pelvis.
2. EBP = early blood pool.
3. This photon-deficient area could be caused by a metallic coin.
4. Administered dose = 500-600 MBq.
5. Phases:
   (i) arterial phase – for 1 minute post injection.
   (ii) blood pool phase – 3 minutes post injection.
   (iii) delayed/static phase – 2-4 hours post injection.

Question 9

1. This is a sagittal T1 W MRI of the cervical spine.
2. A = cerebellar tonsil.
3. B = fourth ventricle.
4. C = clivus.
5. C is of high signal as it contains marrow fat.

Question 10

1. A = left levator ani muscle.
2. B = right sartorius muscle.
3. C = left femoral artery.
4. Total sequencing time = number of excitations × TR × number of phase-encoding steps.
5. T1 W: TE, 30 ms; TR, 300–800 ms.

Question 11

1. This is an MRCP.
2. Sequence: heavily T2 W HASTE
3. Gadolinium is not required.
4. A = fundus of gallbladder.
5. B = left hepatic duct.

Question 12

1. A = cuboid.
2. B = a sesamoid bone.
3. B commonly lies within the tendon of flexor hallucis brevis.
4. The centering point for this view is the cubo-navicular region.
5. C = medial cuneiform.

Question 13

1. This is an occipitofrontal view of the skull with between 10 and 20° of tube angulation. The angulation is assessed by the position of the petrous ridge in relation to the middle of the orbits.
2. A = lambda.
3. B = floor of the sella turcica.
4. C = left inferior turbinate.
5. The pterygopalatine fossa is a posterior relation of the maxillary antrum.

Question 14

1. A = articular tubercle.
2. B = articular disc.
3. C = mandibular condyle.
4. The mouth is open. The position of the condyle is shifted anteriorly to lie against the articular tubercle.
5. The lateral pterygoid muscle is attached to B.

Question 15

1. This image demonstrates that the patient is markedly rotated to the left. The thoracic spinous processes are closer to the medial end of the right clavicle and not equally distant from the medial ends of both clavicles, as in a correctly positioned patient.
2. A = medial border of the right scapula.
3. B = sternoclavicular joint (synovial joint).
4. C = descending thoracic aorta.
5. 65 kV.

Question 16

1. A = right interlobar artery.
2. The interlobar artery may measure 16 mm in men and 15 mm in women.
3. (i) B = hilar point.
   (ii) The hilar point is where the superior pulmonary vein crosses the descending pulmonary artery and the angle between the vessels is known as the hilar angle.
   (iii) The hilar angle normally measures 120°.
4. C = right pericardiophrenic fat pad.
5. D = transverse (minor) fissure.

Question 17

1. This is an LPO/RAO.
2. Contraindications:
   (i) acute respiratory tract infection.
   (ii) poor respiratory reserve.
3 Complications:
   (i) slight impairment in respiratory function – drop in SaO_2 during the procedure and a fall in FEV_1 and FVC at 4 hours.
   (ii) bronchospasm.
4. A = anterior segmental bronchus of left upper lobe.
5. B = inferior lingular segmental bronchus.

Question 18

1. This is a wrist arthrogram.
2. 2-4 ml of contrast is injected into the dorsal aspect of the wrist distal to the midpoint of the distal end of the radius.
3. A = volar radial recess.
4. B = ulnar styloid recess.
5. The normal intercarpal distance = 2 mm (on average).

Question 19

1. This is a barium swallow.
   Indications:
   - (i) dysphagia.
   - (ii) pain.
   - (iii) assessment of tracheooesophageal fistula in a child – a non-ionic agent is preferable.
   - (iv) assessment of the site of perforation – it is essential that a water-soluble contrast medium is used, e.g. LOCM.
2. 100% w/v barium is routinely used.
3. Contraindications: aspiration, perforated viscus.
4. Indentation A is caused by an aberrant right subclavian artery.
5. B = anterior border of the humerus.

Question 20

1. Normal variant: right pelvicalyceal and ureteric duplication.
2. Duplex variant occurs in approximately 0.3% of the population.
3. A = infundibulum of left lower pole calyx.
4. B = right fovea capitis.
5. Contraindications:
   - (i) renal obstruction.
   - (ii) postlaparotomy.
   - (iii) children.
   - (iv) abdominal aortic aneurysm.
   - (v) presence of a colostomy.
   - (vi) renal trauma.

Exam 4

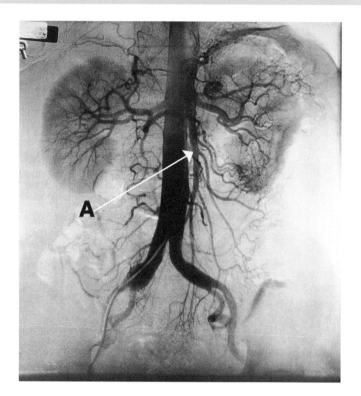

Question 1

1. What is this investigation?
2. What type of catheter is commonly used?
3. What is the normal variant shown?
4. In what percentage does this variant normally occur?
5. Name structure A.

Exam 4

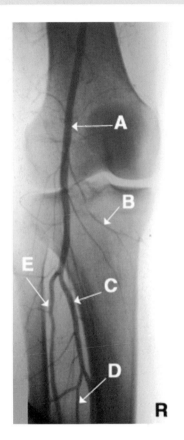

Question 2

1. Name structure A.
2. Name structure B.
3. Name structure C.
4. Name structure D.
5. Name structure E.

Exam 4

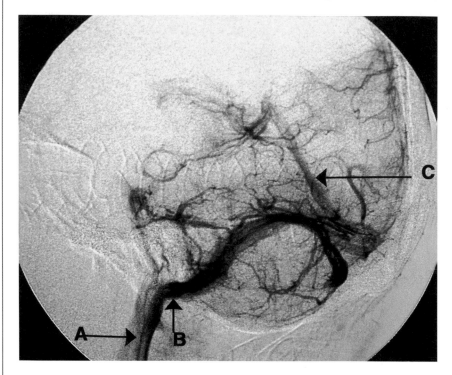

Question 3

1. Name structure A.
2. Name structure B.
3. Which cranial nerves exit the skull with structure A?
4. Name structure C.
5. Which transverse sinus is normally larger and why?

Exam 4

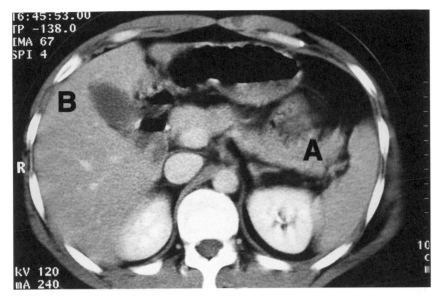

Question 4

1. Name structure A.
2. In which ligament does structure A lie?
3. Give the normal approximate Hounsfield units for:
   (i)   fat.
   (ii) muscle.
4. What segment of the liver does B indicate?
5. What is the approximate rate and volume of contrast given in a 'typical CT scan of the abdomen'?

Exam 4

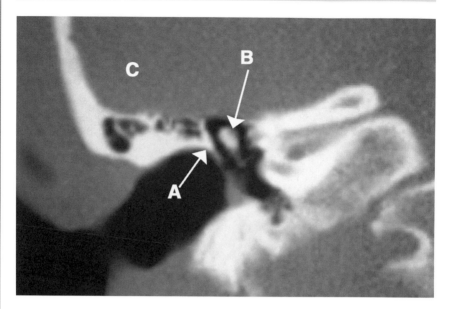

Question 5

1. Name structure A.
2. Name structure B.
3. Which of the ossicles lies most posterior?
4. Name structure C.
5. Name other methods of imaging this area.

Exam 4

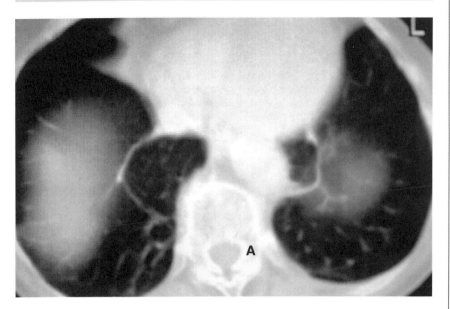

Question 6

1. What normal variant is demonstrated?
2. What is the incidence of this normal variant?
3. Name structure A.
4. Which algorithm is used for this investigation?
5. How does this investigation differ from HRCT?

Exam 4

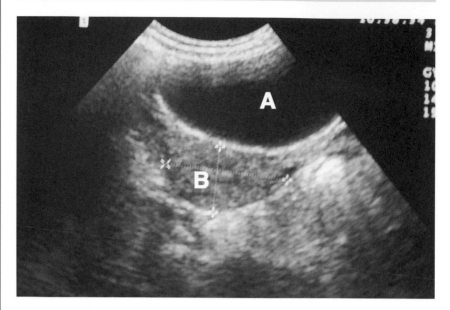

Question 7

1. What frequency transducer is commonly used for this investigation?
2. What is A and why should it be distended?
3. Name structure B.
4. What are the normal dimensions for structure B?
5. What kind of transducer is used for transvaginal scanning?

Exam 4

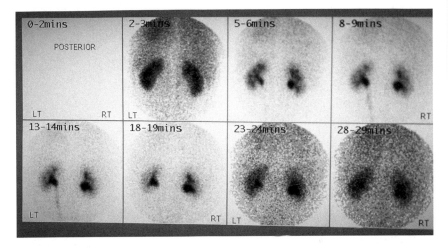

Question 8

1. What is this study?
2. Name three radiopharmaceuticals used for this type of study.
3. Which of these agents is optimal for patients with poor renal function?
4. What other adjuvant medication can be administered during the study and why?
5. Which radiopharmaceutical agent optimally demonstrates renal scarring?

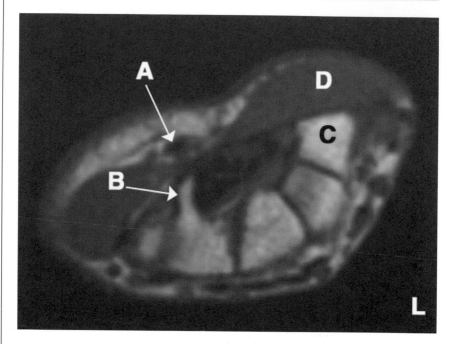

Question 9

1. What is this investigation?
2. Name structure A.
3. Name structure B.
4. Name structure C.
5. Name structure D.

Exam 4

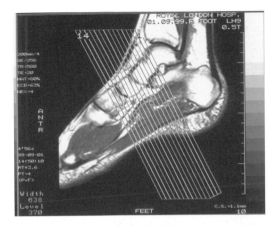

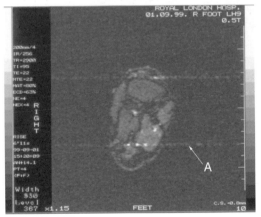

Question 10

1. What is this investigation?
2. What evidence is there that this is a specific sequence?
3. Why is this sequence performed?
4. What is the cause of line A?
5. In which encoding direction does line A normally occur?

Exam 4

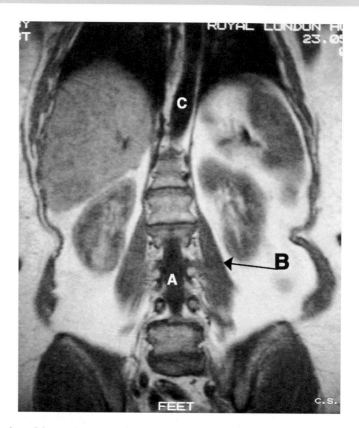

Question 11

1. What is this investigation?
2. Name structure A.
3. Name structure B.
4. Name structure C.
5. What effects do the following manoeuvres have on signal intensity:
   - (i) increasing TR?
   - (ii) increasing TE?

Exam 4

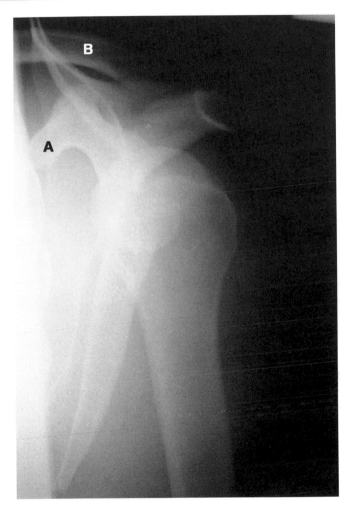

Question 12

1. What view has been taken?
2. Name a specific indication for performing this view.
3. What is the centering point?
4. Name structure A.
5. Name structure B.

Exam 4

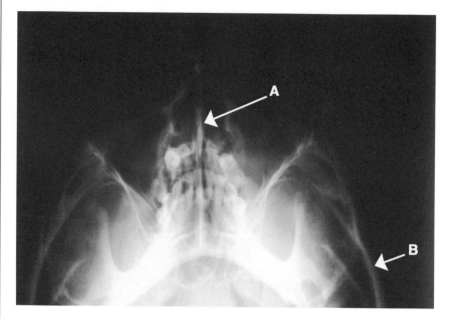

Question 13

1. What view is demonstrated?
2. What is the centering point?
3. Name structure A.
4. Name structure B.
5. What is the radiographic baseline?

Exam 4

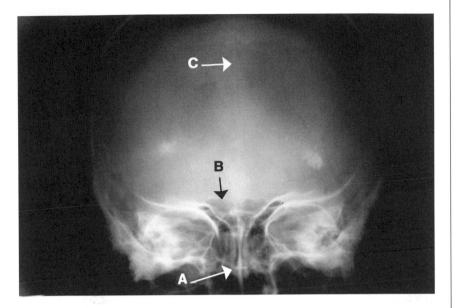

Question 14

1. What is the normal variant demonstrated?
2. Name structure A.
3. Name structure B.
4. Name structure C.
5. In approximately what percentage of the population does C occur?

Exam 4

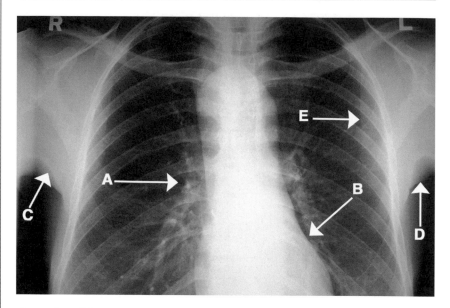

Question 15

1. What normal variant is demonstrated?
2. Name structure A.
3. Name structure B.
4. Name structures C and D.
5. Name structure E.

Exam 4

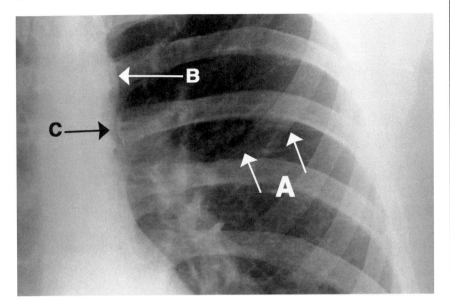

Question 16

1. Name structure A.
2. What does structure A divide?
3. Name structure B.
4. What vessel sometimes gives rise to an aortic nipple?
5. Name structure C.

Exam 4

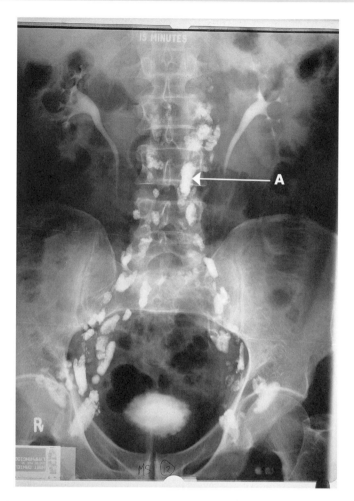

Question 17

1. What is this investigation?
2. Give two contraindications.
3. At what stage is the IVU normally performed following the lymphan-giogram?
4. Name structure A.
5. At what level does the cisterna chyli lie?

Exam 4

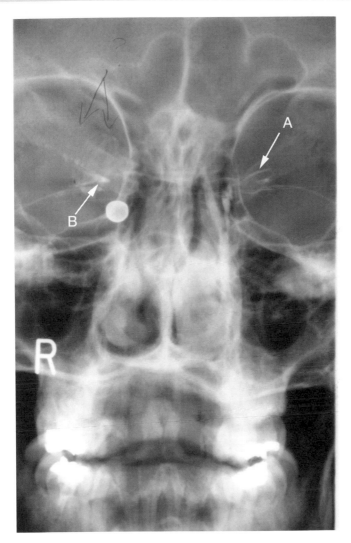

Question 18

1. What is this investigation?
2. What contrast may be used?
3. Where is contrast injected?
4. Name structure A.
5. Name structure B.

Exam 4

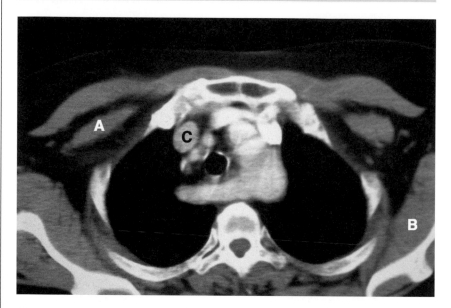

Question 19

1. What normal variant is demonstrated in this investigation?
2. In what percentage of individuals does this normal variant occur?
3. Name structure A.
4. Name structure B.
5. Name structure C.

Exam 4

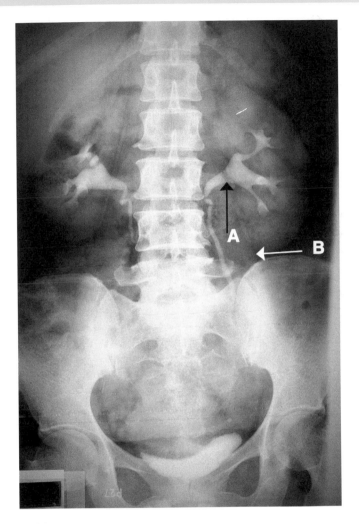

Question 20

1. What is this investigation?
2. Describe the type of contrast used for this investigation and give the administered volume.
3. Name structure A.
4. Is this an adequate film? Give your reasons.
5. Name structure B. Where does it insert?

Question 1

1. This is a flush aortogram (DSA).
2. A pigtail catheter is normally used.
3. Bilateral accessory renal arteries are shown.
4. Accessory renal arteries occur in 25% of normal individuals.
5. A = superior mesenteric artery.

Question 2

1. A = right popliteal artery.
2. B = right medial inferior genicular artery.
3. C = right tibioperoneal trunk.
4. D = right peroneal artery.
5. E = right anterior tibial artery.

Question 3

1. A = internal jugular vein.
2. B = jugular bulb.
3. Cranial nerves IX, X and XI exit the skull with the internal jugular vein.
4. C = straight sinus.
5. The right transverse sinus is normally larger as it receives the major part of the superior sagittal sinus.

Question 4

1. A = tail of the pancreas.
2. The tail of the pancreas normally lies in the lienorenal ligament.
3. Hounsfield unit:
    (i)   fat = −80.
    (ii) muscle = +50.
4. B = segment 5.
5. 100 ml of contrast given at 2-4 ml per second is appropriate in a typical CT scan.

Question 5

1. A = scutum.
2. B = incudomalleolar complex.
3. The incus lies most posterior.
4. C = temporal lobe in the middle cranial fossa.
5. Both MRI and plain film tomography provide additional methods of imaging this area.

Question 6

1. This image demonstrates bilateral inferior accessory fissures.
2. Inferior accessory fissures are seen in 8% of PA chest X-rays and are found in 45% of postmortem examinations. They are also called Twining's lines.
3. A = left pedicle.
4. A soft tissue algorithm has been used for this investigation.
5. Bone algorithms are used in HRCT.

Question 7

1. A 3.5 MHz transducer is frequently used for transabdominal pelvic scanning.
2. A = bladder. The bladder should be full as it provides an acoustic window to image the structures immediately behind it, i.e. the uterus and ovaries.
3. B = uterus.
4. The normal dimensions of the uterus are 8×5 cm.
5. For transvaginal scanning a 7.5 MHz rotary scanner is frequently used.

Question 8

1. This is dynamic renal scintigraphy.
2. (i) ^{99m}Tc-MAG$_3$.
   (ii) ^{99m}Tc-DTPA.
   (iii) ^{123}I Hippuran.
3. ^{99m}Tc-MAG$_3$ is the agent of choice in patients with poor renal function.
4. (i) Frusemide may be administered to confirm or refute renal obstruction.
   (ii) Captopril may be administered to identify patients with renal vascular hypertension.
5. ^{99m}Tc-DMSA is the agent of choice in the detection of renal scarring.

Question 9

1. This is an axial MRI of the left wrist.
2. A = left ulnar artery.
3. B = left hook of hammate.
4. C = left trapezium.
5. D = left abductor pollicis brevis muscle.

Question 10

1. This is an axial STIR sequence of the right ankle.
2. 'IR' (inversion recovery) is marked on the image.
3. STIR sequences are performed for fat suppression.
4. Line A is due to pulsation artefact secondary to plantar vessels.
5. Line A occurs in the phase-encoding direction.

Question 11

1. This is a coronal T1–weighted MRI of the abdomen.
2. A = thecal sac.
3. B = left psoas muscle.
4. C = descending aorta.
5. (i) Increasing TR – increases signal.
   (ii) Increasing TE – decreases signal.

Question 12

1. This is a Y-view of the scapula.
2. A specific indication is an assessment of the dislocation of the shoulder.
3. Centering point: head of the humerus through the medial border of the scapula at the level of the 4th thoracic vertebra.
4. A = coracoid process.
5. B = clavicle.

Question 13

1. This is an occipitomental 30° (OM 30).
2. Centering point: midline through the vertex to the level of the lower orbital margin.
3. A = nasal septum.
4. B = left zygomatic arch.
5. The radiographic baseline is a line drawn from the external auditory meatus to the outer canthus of the eye.

Question 14

1. Choroid plexus calcification in the lateral ventricles is demonstrated.
2. A = floor of the sella turcica.
3. B = right frontal sinus.
4. C = calcification within the falx cerebri.
5. Calcification in the falx occurs in approximately 7% of the population.

Question 15

1. A right side aortic arch is demonstrated.
2. A = right hilar point – where the upper lobe vein crosses the descending pulmonary artery.
3. B = left atrial appendage.
4. C = anterior axillary skinfold, D = posterior axillary skinfold.
5. E = medial border of the left scapula.

Question 16

1. A = left horizontal fissure.
2. The left horizontal fissure divides the left upper lobe from the lingular segment.
3. B = aortic knuckle.
4. A left superior intercostal vein sometimes gives rise to an aortic nipple.
5. C = left costovertebral joint.

Question 17

1. This is a lymphangiogram.
2. Contraindications:
   (i)   left-to-right shunt.
   (ii) this examination should not be performed within 3 weeks of radio-therapy or chemotherapy.
   (iii) local sepsis at the injection site.
   (iv) severe respiratory disease.
3. The IVU is normally performed 24 hours postinjection.
4. A = left para aortic lymph nodes.
5. The cisterna chyli lies at L1.

Question 18

1. This is a bilateral dacrocystogram.
2. Contrast used: non–ionic/Lipiodol (0.5–2 ml per side).
3. Contrast is injected into the inferior canaliculus.
4. A = left superior canaliculus.
5. B = right common canaliculus.

Question 19

1. This image demonstrates an aberrant right subclavian artery.
2. An aberrant right subclavian artery occurs in 0.25–1% of the population.
3. A = right pectoralis minor muscle.
4. B = left subscapularis muscle.
5. C = right brachiocephalic vein.

Question 20

1. This is an IVU.
2. Low osmolar contrast medium: 300–350 mg per ml is routinely used. The administered volume = 1 ml per kg body weight.
3. A = vascular impression superimposed over the left renal pelvis.
4. This is an adequate film as the coned area is from the costal margin to the pubic symphysis inclusive. As a result, the entire renal tract can be visualized on this one film.
5. B = left psoas muscle. This inserts into the lesser trochanter of the femur.

Exam 5

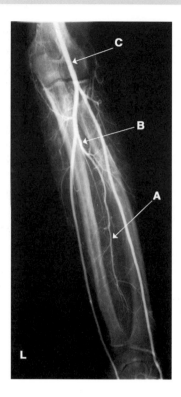

Question 1

1. What is this investigation?
2. Name two indications for this investigation.
3. Name structure A.
4. Name structure B.
5. Name structure C.

Exam 5

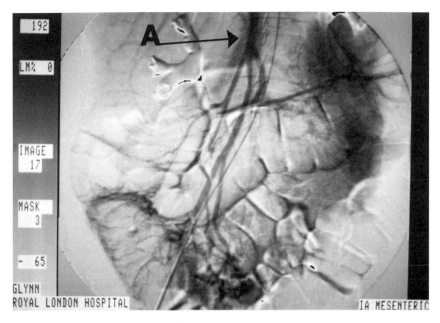

Question 2

1. What is this investigation?
2. Name structure A.
3. Which structure joins A to form the portal vein?
4. What proportion of the total blood flow to the liver is typically supplied by the portal vein?
5. What is the normal relationship of A to the superior mesenteric artery (SMA) and what does the opposite relationship indicate?

Exam 5

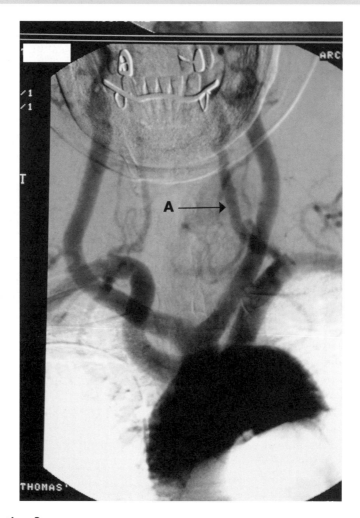

Question 3

1. What is this investigation?
2. What is the normal variant demonstrated?
3. Name structure A.
4. In what percentage of the population is the left vertebral artery dominant?
5. What is the most common anatomical variant of the great vessels?

Exam 5

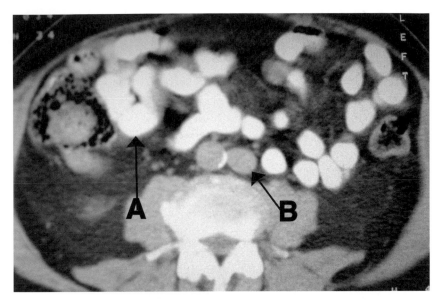

Question 4

1. Name structure A.
2. Give the typical concentration of oral contrast used in CT.
3. How long before scanning should oral contrast be given to the patient for the following investigations:
   (i)   large bowel?
   (ii) small bowel?
4. Name structure B.
5. What is the normal maximum calibre of B?

Exam 5

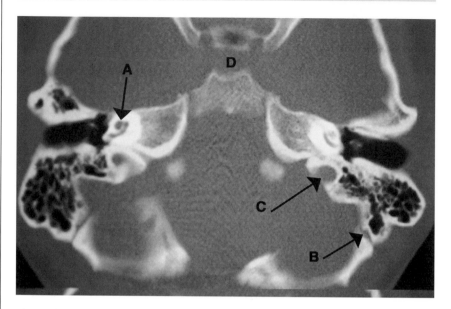

Question 5

1. Name structure A.
2. Name structure B.
3. Which nerves accompany the vessel that passes through structure C?
4. Which structure lies at D?
5. Is spiral or conventional axial scanning performed in CT of the head?

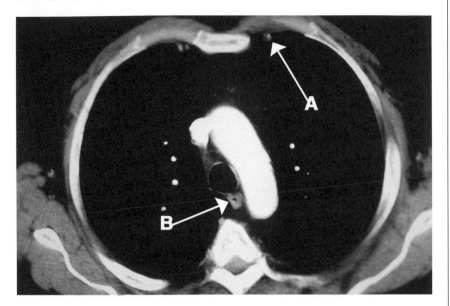

Question 6

1. Name structure A.
2. Name structure B.
3. At what level does structure B pierce the diaphragm?
4. How are CT numbers calculated?
5. Give an approximate CT number for the following:
   - (i)   fat.
   - (ii)   muscle.
   - (iii) water.

Exam 5

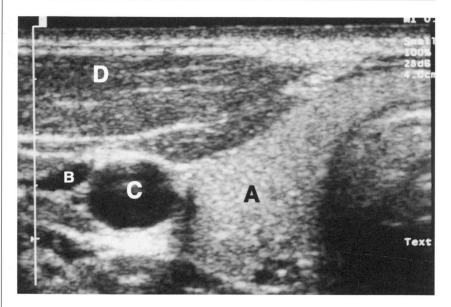

Question 7

1. Name structure A.
2. Name structure B.
3. Name structure C.
4. Name structure D.
5. At what vertebral level does C bifurcate?

Exam 5

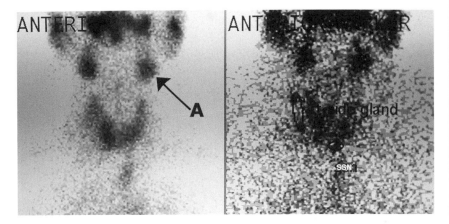

Question 8

1. What is this investigation?
2. Which radionuclide is used and what is the administered dose?
3. Name structure A.
4. What do the initials 'SSN' indicate?
5. Which radionuclide is usually used for skin markers?

Exam 5

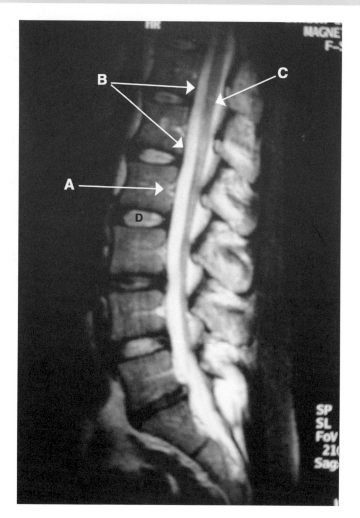

Question 9

1. What is this investigation?
2. Name structure A.
3. Name structure B.
4. Name structure C.
5. Why is structure D of high signal?

Exam 5

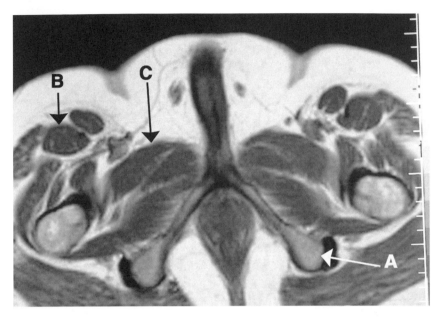

Question 10

1. Name structure A.
2. Name structure B.
3. Name structure C.
4. What signal does 'fluid' return on T1 W MRI?
5. Name three structures that are black (low signal) on both T1 W and T2 W MRI.

Exam 5

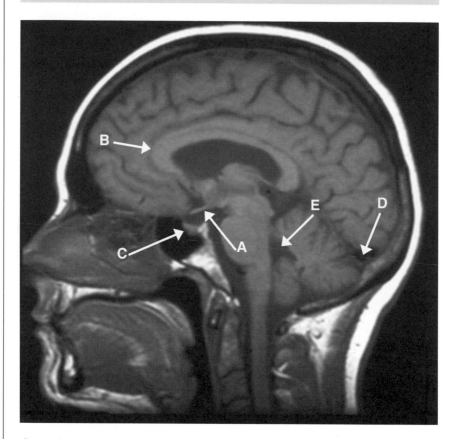

Question 11

1. Name structure A.
2. Name structure B.
3. Name structure C.
4. Name structure D.
5. Describe the openings within structure E.

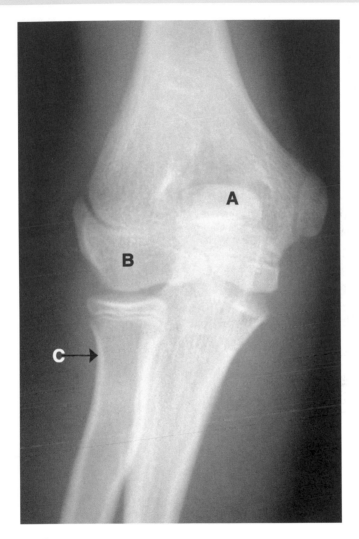

Question 12

1. Name structure A.
2. Name structure B.
3. Name structure C.
4. What is the approximate age of this patient?
5. In what order do the ossification centres of the elbow appear?

Exam 5

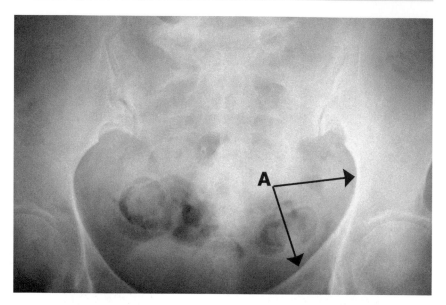

Question 13

1. What normal variant is demonstrated?
2. What passes through this normal variant?
3. In which gender is this normal variant usually seen?
4. Name structure A.
5. Is AP or PA better for visualizing the SI joints and why?

Exam 5

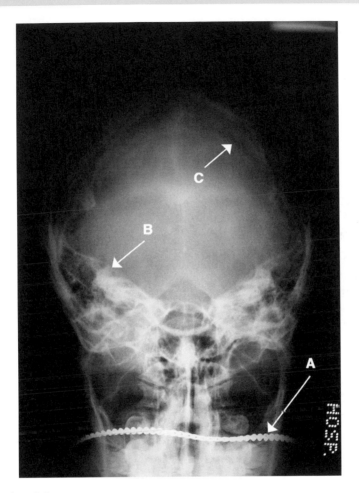

Question 14

1. What view is demonstrated?
2. Name structure A.
3. Name structure B.
4. Name structure C.
5. Is this a routine skull view and if not, how do you know?

Exam 5

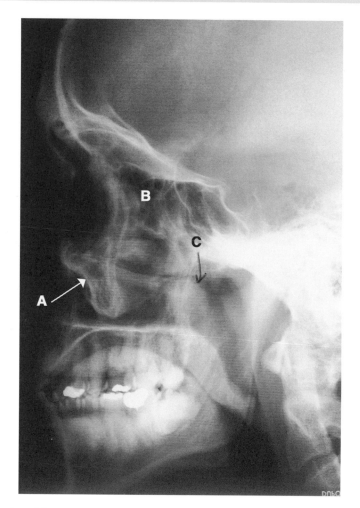

Question 15

1. Name structure A.
2. Name structure B.
3. Name the high-density area indicated by arrow C.
4. What is the cause of structure C?
5. Which bones are the nasal conchae a part of?

Exam 5

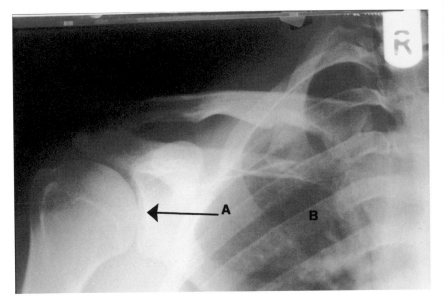

Question 16

1. What normal variant is shown?
2. What structure is attached to this normal variant?
3. Name structure A.
4. What is the normal acromiohumeral distance?
5. Name structure B.

Exam 5

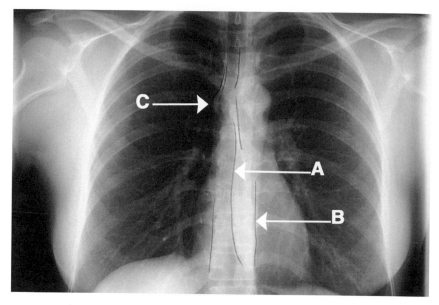

Question 17

1. What is line A?
2. What is line B?
3. What is the normal width of line B?
4. Which structure is situated at point C?
5. Under what physiological circumstances does structure C increase in size?

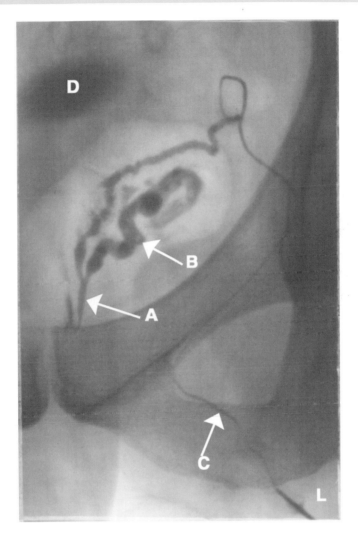

Question 18

1. What is this examination?
2. Name structure A.
3. Name structure B.
4. Name structure C.
5. Name structure D.

Exam 5

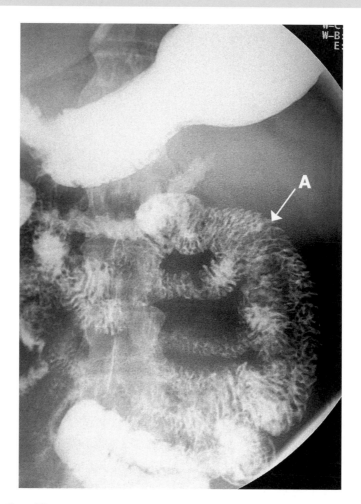

Question 19

1. What is this investigation?
2. What volume and concentration of barium should be used in this investigation?
3. Name structure A.
4. What is the maximum diameter of A?
5. Name two methods of optimally visualising the terminal ileum in this study.

Exam 5

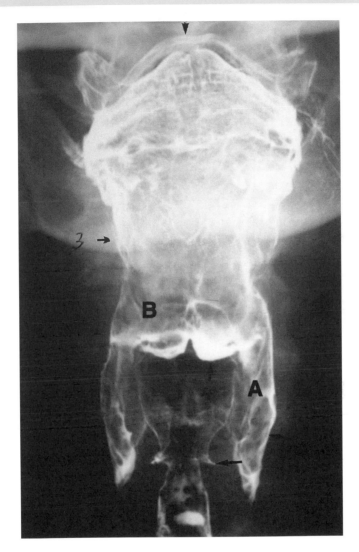

Question 20

1. Name structure A.
2. Name structure B.
3. Which structure forms:
   (i)   the medial wall of A?
   (ii) the lateral wall of A?
4. Which contrast agent has been used here?
5. At which vertebra levels do the (i) hyoid and (ii) cricoid lie?

Question 1

1. This is a left brachial arteriogram.
2. Indications:
    (i) investigation of arterial ischaemia.
    (ii) trauma.
    (iii) investigation of a mass.
    (iv) arteriovenous malformation.
3. A = left posterior interosseous artery.
4. B = left common interosseous artery.
5. C = left brachial artery.

Question 2

1. This is a late phase (venous-phase) superior mesenteric artery angiogram (DSA).
2. A = superior mesenteric vein (SMV).
3. The splenic vein joins with the SMV to form the portal vein.
4. Approximately 75% of the blood supply to the liver is supplied by the portal vein.
5. Normally the SMV is to the right of the SMA. If the SMV is to the left, this indicates a malrotation.

Question 3

1. This is an IA DSA arch aortogram.
2. The normal variant demonstrated is common origin of the common carotid artery.
3. A = left vertebral artery.
4. The left vertebral artery is dominant in 60% of the population.
5. The left vertebral artery arising directly from the arch of the aorta is the most common normal variant of the great vessels.

Question 4

1. A = a loop of small bowel containing contrast.
2. The typical concentration of oral contrast = 3% gastrograffin.
3. (i) large bowel – contrast is usually given 90 minutes before the scan.
    (ii) small bowel – contrast is given 30-60 minutes prior to scanning.
4. B = descending aorta.
5. The normal maximum calibre of B = 3 cm.

Question 5

1. A = right cochlea.
2. B = left lambdoid suture.
3. C = left jugular foramen. Cranial nerves IX, X and XI accompany the internal jugular vein through this foramen.
4. Pituitary gland.
5. CT scanning of the head is usually performed with a conventional axial technique.

Question 6

1. A = left internal thoracic artery.
2. B = oesophagus.
3. The oesophagus pierces the diaphragm at T10.
4. CT number $= 1000 \times (u_T - u_{water}/u_{water})$
   where u_T = attenuation coefficient of the tissue in question and u_{water} = the attenuation coefficient of water.
5. CT number:
   (i)   fat = −80.
   (ii)   muscle = +50.
   (iii)   water = 0.

Question 7

1. A = right lobe of the thyroid gland.
2. B = right internal jugular vein.
3. C = right common carotid artery.
4. D = right sternocleidomastoid muscle.
5. The common carotid artery bifurcates at C3–4.

Question 8

1. This is a radionuclide thyroid scan.
2. Radionuclide: ^{99m}Tc-pertechnetate. Administered dose = 60 MBq.
3. A = left submandibular gland.
4. 'SSN' indicates position of the suprasternal notch.
5. Skin markers are usually indicated by the use of radioactive cobalt-57.

Question 9

1. This is a sagittal T2 W MRI of the lumbosacral spine.
2. A = basivertebral vein of L2.
3. B = posterior longitudinal ligament.
4. C = conus medullaris.
5. D = nucleus pulposus – this returns a high signal due to the presence of fluid within the disc.

Question 10

1. A = left ischial tuberosity.
2. B = right rectus femoris muscle.
3. C = right pectineus muscle.
4. Fluid appears black on T1 W imaging.
5. Structures appearing black on both T1 W and T2 W imaging: tendons, ligaments, cortical bone and air.

Question 11

1. A = optic chiasm.
2. B = genu of the corpus callosum.
3. C = pituitary gland.
4. D = transverse sinus.
5. E = cavity of the 4th ventricle. The 4th ventricle contains three foramina by which CSF drains – the midline foramen of Magendie and the two lateral foramina of Lushka.

Question 12

1. A = ossification centre of the olecranon.
2. B = ossification centre of the capitellum.
3. C = radial neck.
4. The patient is approximately 9–10 years old.
5. Order of ossification at the elbow: capitellum, radial head, internal epi-condyle, trochlea, olecranon process and lateral epicondyle (CRITOL).

Question 13

1. A paraglenoid fossa (or preauricular sulcus) is demonstrated.
2. The superior gluteal artery usually passes through this fossa.
3. This variant is usually identifiable in females only.
4. A = iliopectineal line.
5. A PA image is better for demonstrating the SI as the diverging X-ray beam traverses the plane of the joints themselves.

Question 14

1. This is a Towne's view.
2. A = metallic artefact in the form of a necklace.
3. B = right petrous ridge.
4. C = left lambdoid suture.
5. This is not a routine skull view. Towne's views are performed in the trauma setting.

Question 15

1. A = zygoma.
2. B = sphenoid sinus.
3. C = nasal pseudotumour.
4. The nasal pseudotumour is a composite density consisting of the inferior nasal concha and the coronoid process of the mandible.
5. The superior and middle conchae arise from the ethmoid bone. The inferior concha is a bone in its own right.

Question 16

1. The normal variant demonstrated is a rhomboid fossa on the infero-medial aspect of the clavicle.
2. The rhomboid fossa is formed from insertion of the costoclavicular ligament.
3. A = right glenoid fossa.
4. The normal acromiohumeral distance = 6–7 mm.
5. B = right posterior 5th rib.

Question 17

1. A = azygo-oesophageal line.
2. B = left paravertebral line.
3. The left paravertebral line can measure up to 1 cm in width.
4. The azygous vein usually lies at point C.
5. The diameter of the azygous vein increases in the supine position, in expiration and when performing a reverse Valsalva manoeuvre.

Question 18

1. This is a vasogram.
2. A = left ejaculatory duct.
3. B = left seminal vesicle.
4. C = left vas deferens.
5. D = contrast within the bladder.

Question 19

1. This is a barium follow-through.
2. 300–600 ml of 100% w/v barium should be given.
3. A = jejunum.
4. The maximum diameter of the jejunum = 3.5 cm.
5. The terminal ileum is better visualized using:
   (i) focal compression pad.
   (ii) pneumocolon technique.

Question 20

1. A = left piriform fossa.
2. B = right vallecula.
3. (i)   The medial wall is formed from the aryepiglottic fold.
   (ii)   The lateral wall is formed from the thyrohyoid membrane.
4. Barium has been used here.
5. (i) Hyoid bone – C3 and (ii) cricoid cartilage – C6.

Exam 6

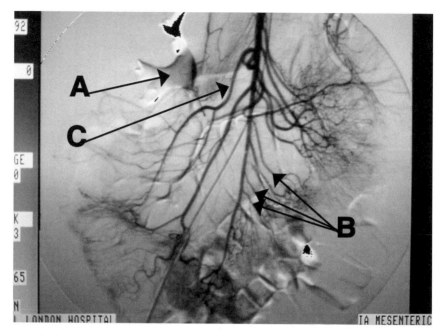

Question 1

1. Name structure A.
2. Name structure B.
3. Name structure C.
4. What pharmacological agent is used in this study and why?
5. Is breath holding required and why?

Exam 6

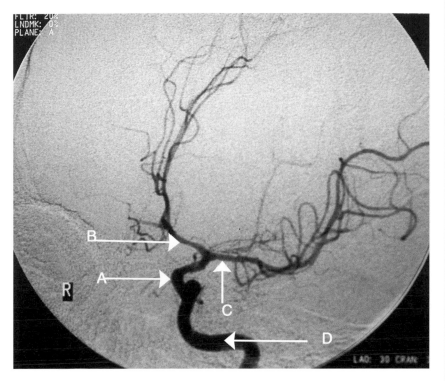

Question 2

1. What investigation is this?
2. Through which structure does A commonly traverse?
3. Name structure B.
4. Name structure C.
5. Which part of the artery does structure D represent?

Exam 6

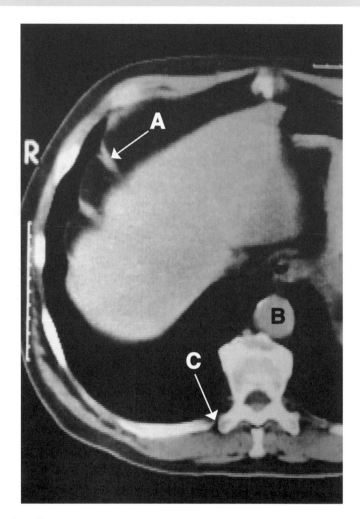

Question 3

1. Name structure A.
2. Can structure A be seen on ultrasound?
3. Why is breath holding normally required for abdominal CT scanning?
4. Name structure B.
5. What type of joint is C?

Exam 6

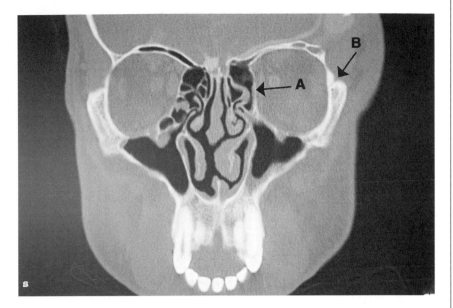

Question 4

1. What is this investigation?
2. What are typical window widths and levels for this investigation?
3. Name structure A.
4. Which bones form the nasal septum?
5. Name structure B.

Exam 6

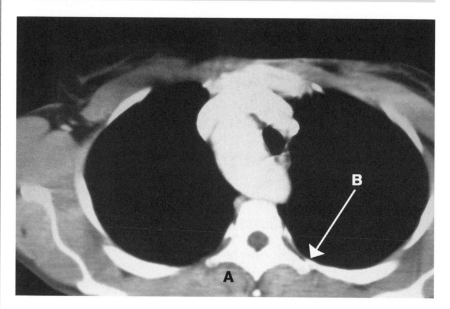

Question 5

1. What is the normal variant shown?
2. Approximately how much contrast and at what rate is it administered for this investigation?
3. Name structure A.
4. Name structure B.
5. What would be appropriate window settings for this image?

Exam 6

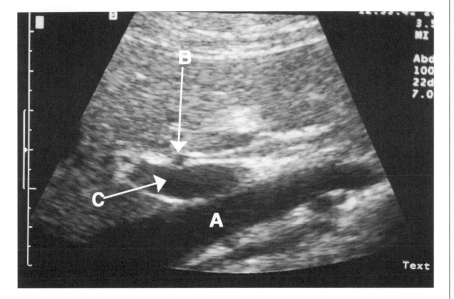

Question 6

1. What is the imaging plane of this scan?
2. Name structure A.
3. Name structure B.
4. Name structure C.
5. What is the common patient preparation for an upper abdominal ultrasound scan?

Exam 6

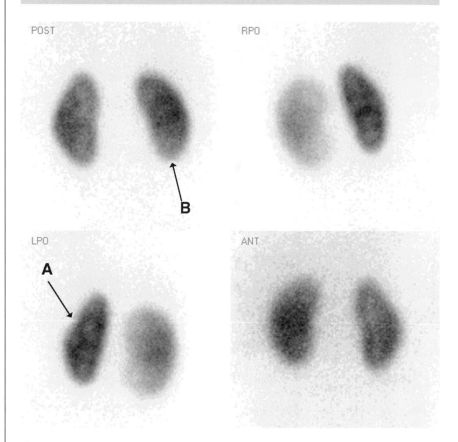

Question 7

1. What is this investigation and name two agents that may be used?
2. Name three indications for this investigation.
3. What does A indicate?
4. Name structure B.
5. How is relative renal function calculated?

Exam 6

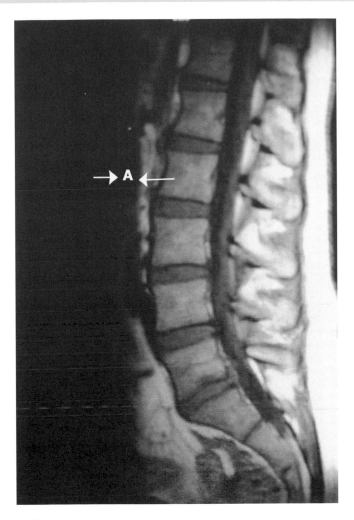

Question 8

1. What sequence is this?
2. Name structure A.
3. What type of coil is used for this investigation?
4. Describe two benefits of using a local coil.
5. Name two indications for the use of gadolinium when imaging the lumbar spine.

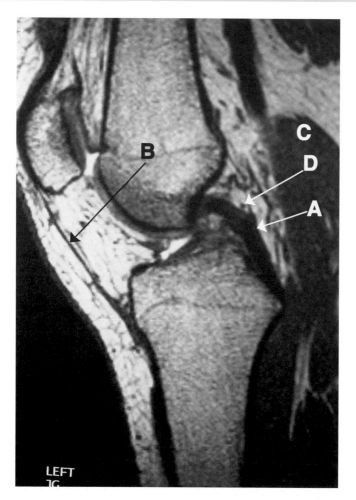

LEFT
TG

Question 9

1. Name structure A.
2. Name structure B.
3. Name structure C.
4. Name structure D.
5. Can patients with the following implants undergo MRI:
   - (i)   knee prostheses?
   - (ii) cardiac valve?
   - (iii) permanent pacemaker?

Exam 6

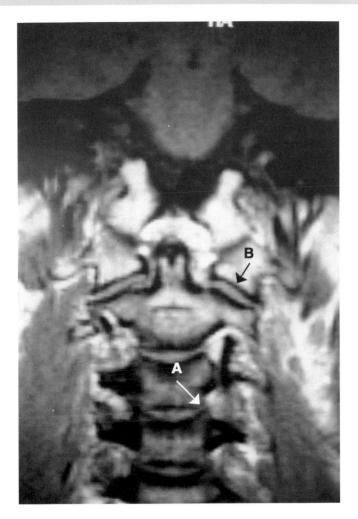

Question 10

1. What sequence has been performed?
2. Name joint A.
3. What type of joint is A?
4. Name joint B.
5. Name the ligaments attached to the tip of the odontoid process.

Exam 6

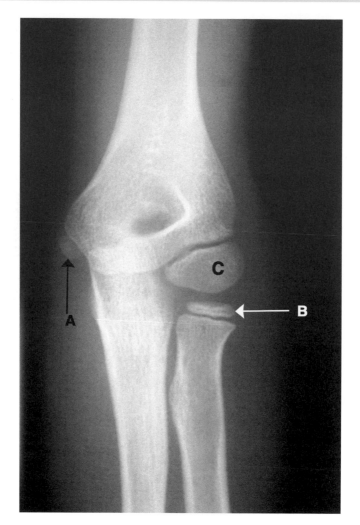

Question 11

1. What is this view?
2. Name structure A.
3. Name structure B.
4. Name structure C.
5. What is the approximate age of this patient?

Exam 6

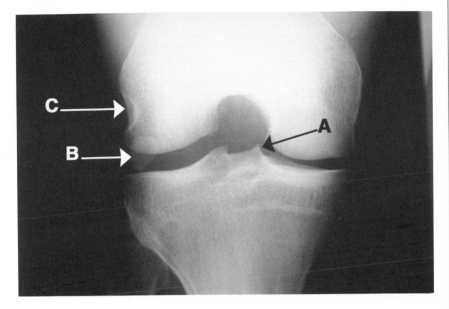

Question 12

1. What view has been performed?
2. Name structure A.
3. Name structure B.
4. What tendon does B lie in?
5. What structure causes the notch C?

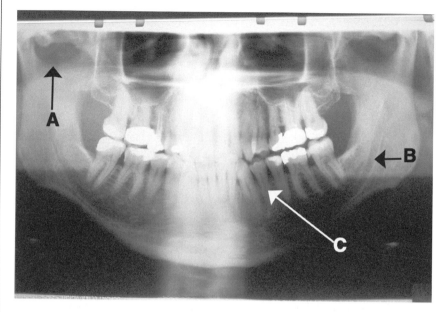

Question 13

1. What is this investigation?
2. Name structure A.
3. Name structure B.
4. Name structure C.
5. What other view is routinely performed for imaging the mandible?

Exam 6

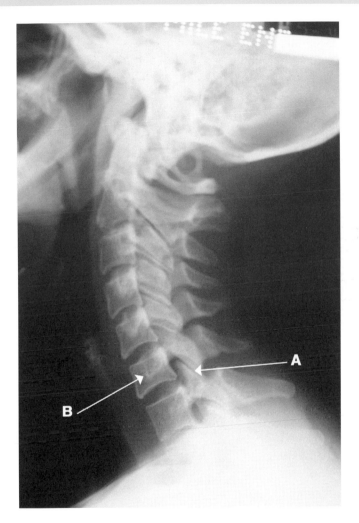

Question 14

1. What is the centering point for this view?
2. What is the normal variant shown and what is its aetiology?
3. What structure runs through this normal variant?
4. Name structure A.
5. Name structure B.

Exam 6

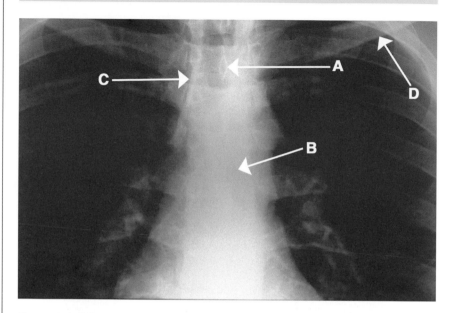

Question 15

1. Name structure A.
2. Name structure B.
3. Name structure C.
4. What is the normal size of structure C?
5. How does bone D ossify and at what age does it undergo ossification?

Exam 6

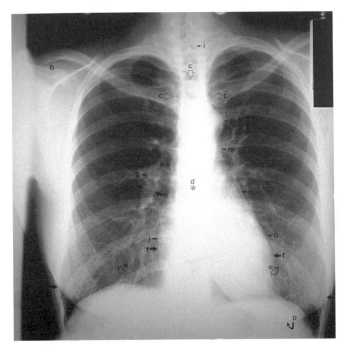

Question 16

1. Using C, how do you judge the rotation of the patient?
2. What structure is represented by arrow P?
3. What does letter F represent?
4. Is this a high or low kV film and how do you know?
5. What is the centering point for a PA chest X-ray.

Exam 6

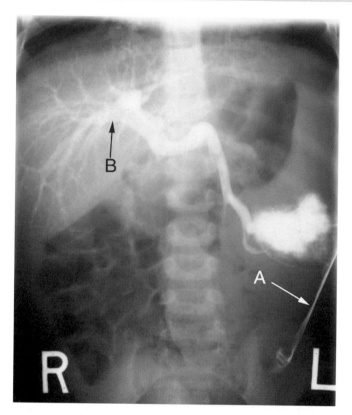

Question 17

1. What is this investigation?
2. How is contrast administered and at what volume and rate is it introduced?
3. Name structure A.
4. Name structure B.
5. Name three complications of this investigation.

Exam 6

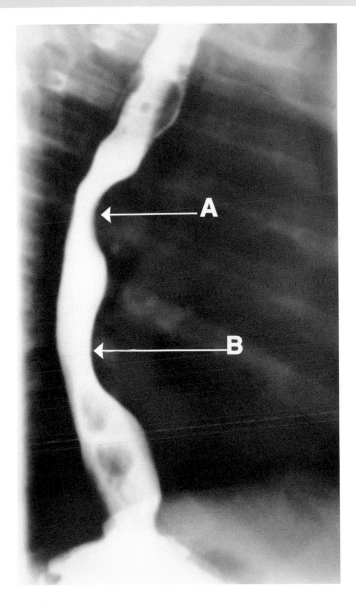

Question 18

1. What is the cause of indentation A?
2. What is the cause of indentation B?
3. At what level does the oesophagus pierce the diaphragm?
4. Which nerves accompany the oesophagus through the diaphragm?
5. Give two contraindications to the use of barium in the study.

Exam 6

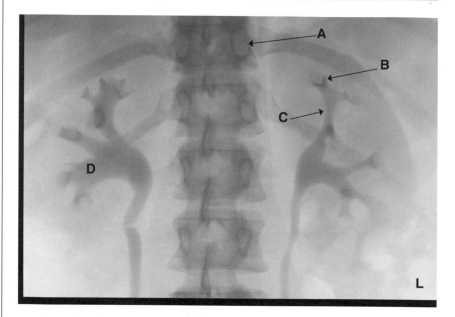

Question 19

1. Name structure A.
2. Name structure B.
3. Name structure C.
4. Name structure D.
5. What is the paediatric contrast dose for such an investigation?

Exam 6

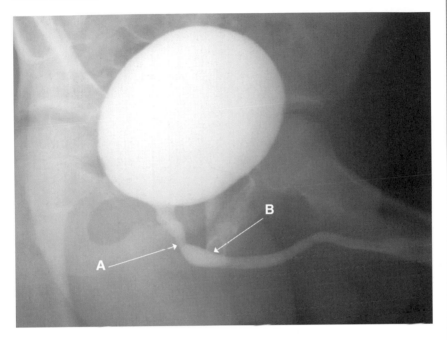

Question 20

1. Name three indications for this investigation.
2. Name two contraindications for this test.
3. What position is shown?
4. Name structure A.
5. Name structure B.

Question 1

1. A = right renal pelvis.
2. B = ileal branches of the superior mesenteric artery.
3. C = right colic artery.
4. Buscopan IV or glucagon IV is administered to reduce bowel movement artefact.
5. Breath holding is essential to reduce movement artefact.

Question 2

1. This is a right internal carotid digital subtraction angiogram.
2. This part of the internal carotid artery traverses the cavernous sinus.
3. B = right anterior cerebral artery.
4. C = right middle cerebral artery.
5. D = petrous part of the right internal carotid artery.

Question 3

1. A = diaphragmatic slips.
2. Diaphragmatic slips are commonly seen on ultrasound.
3. Breath holding is employed to reduce movement artefact.
4. B = descending aorta.
5. C = costotransverse joint (synovial type).

Question 4

1. This is a coronal CT of the paranasal sinuses imaged on bony window settings.
2. Window level = +500, window width = 1500.
3. A = left lamina papyracea.
4. The bony part of the nasal septum is formed from the vomer and the perpendicular plate of the ethmoid bone.
5. B = left frontozygomatic suture.

Question 5

1. A right-sided aortic arch is demonstrated.
2. 90–100 ml of contrast at 2 ml per second with an imaging delay of 30 seconds would be appropriate for computed tomography of the thorax.
3. A = right erector spinae muscle.
4. B = left costotransverse joint.
5. Window settings: window level 40, window width 340–400.

Question 6

1. This is a longitudinal view through the upper abdomen.
2. A = IVC.
3. B = hepatic artery.
4. C = portal vein.
5. The patient should be fasted for 4–6 hours.

Question 7

1. This is a static renal scintogram. Agents: ^{99m}Tc-DMSA, ^{99m}Tc-gluco-heptonate.
2. Indications:
   (i) assessment of individual renal function.
   (ii) assessment of the non-functioning kidney on excretion urography.
   (iii) demonstration of ectopic renal tissue.
   (iv) assessment of reflux nephropathy.
   (v) acute urinary tract infection.
   (vi) renal tumour.
   (vii) demonstration of congenital abnormalities and mass lesions.
3. A indicates a splenic impression.
4. B = lower pole of the right kidney (posterior view).
5. Relative function is calculated from the geometric mean of posterior and anterior computer images. A single posterior image is often used for this makes the assumption that the kidneys are at the same depth.

Question 8

1. This is a T1 W MRI of the lumbosacral spine.
2. A = descending aorta.
3. The patient lies on a surface coil.
4. The benefits of using a local coil are:
   (i) increased signal-to-noise ratio.
   (ii) decreased motion and aliasing artefacts.
5. Gadolinium is used for lumbar spine imaging:
   (i) to distinguish between postoperative fibrosis and disc herniation.
   (ii) to establish whether a space-occupying lesion enhances.

Question 9

1. A = posterior cruciate ligament.
2. B = patellar tendon.
3. C = medial head of gastrocnemius.
4. D = posterior meniscofemoral ligament.
5. (i) Knee prostheses – yes.
   (ii) Cardiac valve – yes.
   (iii) Permanent pacemaker – no.

Question 10

1. This is a coronal T1 W MRI demonstrating the atlantoaxial joint.
2. A = left uncovertebral joint at C3–4.
3. The uncovertebral joint is of the synovial type.
4. B = left lateral atlantoaxial joint.
5. The alar and apical ligaments are attached to the odontoid process.

Question 11

1. This is an AP view of the elbow in a skeletally immature individual.
2. A = ossification centre of the medial epicondyle.
3. B = ossification centre for the head of the radius.
4. C = ossification centre for the capitellum.
5. The patient is approximately 6 years old.

Question 12

1. This is a tunnel view (intercondylar view).
2. A = medial tibial spine.
3. B = fabella.
4. The fabella lies within the tendon of the lateral head of gastrocnemius.
5. C is caused by the popliteus tendon.

Question 13

1. This is an orthopantomogram (OPG)
2. A = right mandibular notch.
3. B = left mandibular canal.
4. C = left lower first premolar.
5. A PA view is also routinely performed for imaging the mandible.

Question 14

1. Centering point = 2.5 cm posterior to the angle of the mandible.
2. The normal variant demonstrated is an arcuate foramen. This is formed by calcification of the posterior atlantooccipital ligament.
3. The vertebral artery runs through the arcuate foramen.
4. A = facet joint of C6–7.
5. B = anterior tubercle of the transverse process of C6.

Question 15

1. A = spinous process of T3.
2. B = left main bronchus.
3. C = right paratracheal stripe.
4. The right paratracheal stripe is normally 3 mm wide.
5. The clavicle ossifies in membrane. It begins to ossify before any other bone in the body, from two centres that appear at the 5th and 6th foetal weeks.

Question 16

1. Rotation: distances of the medial end of the clavicles to the spinous processes should be equally distant.
2. P = left breast shadow.
3. F demonstrates the Mach effect (this is an optical illusion manifest as a lucent line at an air–water interface).
4. This investigation is a low kV chest X-ray – the bones are well seen. This is in contradistinction to a high kV film where lung parenchyma is better visualized at the expense of bony detail.
5. The centering point of a chest X-ray is in the midline at the level of T6.

Question 17

1. This is a splenoportogram.
2. Contrast is introduced via direct puncture of the spleen. 50 ml is injected at about 10 ml per second.
3. A = intraperitoneal leakage of contrast.
4. B = right portal vein.
5. Complications:
    (i) splenic rupture.
    (ii) haemorrhage.
    (iii) infection.
    (iv) perforation of adjacent viscera.

Question 18

1. The aortic arch causes indentation A.
2. The left main bronchus causes indentation B.
3. The oesophagus pierces the diaphragm at T10.
4. The left and right vagus nerves accompany the oesophagus.
5. Contraindications:
    (i) aspiration.
    (ii) perforation.
    (iii) complete bowel obstruction.

Question 19

1. A = left pedicle of T11.
2. B = fornix of left upper pole calyx.
3. C = infundibulum of left upper pole calyx.
4. D = major calyx of right lower pole.
5. Paediatric contrast dose for an IVU = 1 ml per kg.

Question 20

1. Indications: strictures, urethral tears, congenital abnormality, periurethral or prostatic abscess and fistulae of false passages.
2. Contraindications: acute urinary tract infection and recent instrumentation.
3. Position: 30° RAO, with left leg abducted and knee flexed.
4. A = membranous urethra.
5. B = bulbous urethra.

Exam 7

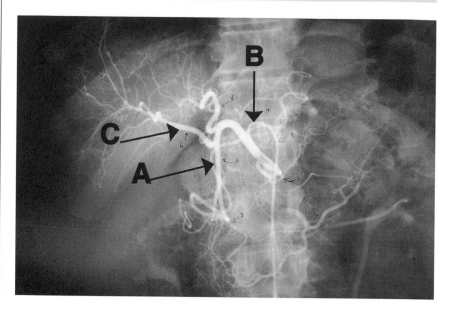

Question 1

1. What is this investigation?
2. Name structure A.
3. Name structure B.
4. Name structure C.
5. In what percentage of normal patients does C arise from the superior mesenteric artery?

Exam 7

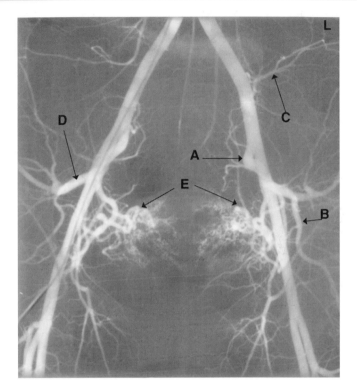

Question 2

1. Name structure A.
2. Name structure B.
3. Name structure C.
4. Name structure D.
5. Name structure E.

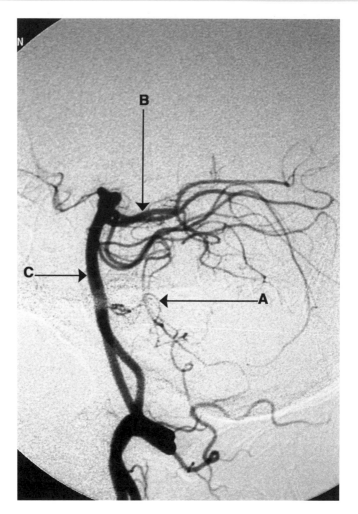

Question 3

1. What is this investigation and what view is demonstrated?
2. To perform this investigation, do two arteries need to be cannulated routinely and why?
3. Name structure A.
4. Name structure B.
5. Which cistern does structure C lie within?

Exam 7

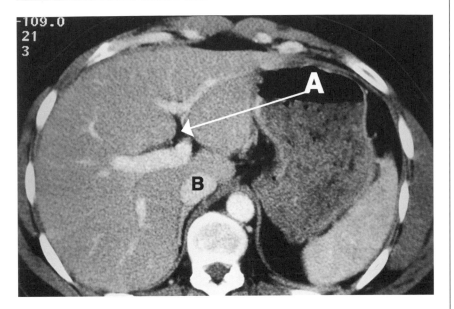

Question 4

1. Name structure A.
2. Which embryological structure traverses A?
3. Name two organs that, when imaged, require water to be given as oral contrast.
4. Is water a positive or negative contrast agent?
5. Name structure B.

Exam 7

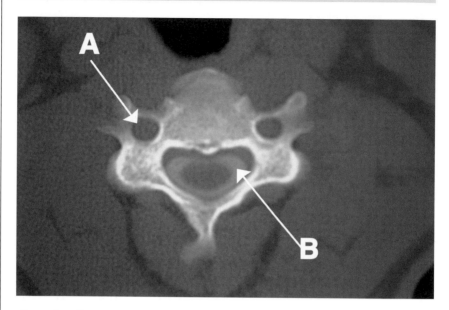

Question 5

1. Name structure A.
2. Which structure runs through A and what is it a branch of?
3. What part of the spinal column is this and give two reasons why you know this.
4. Why is less contrast given in CT myelography compared with conventional myelography?
5. Name structure B.

Exam 7

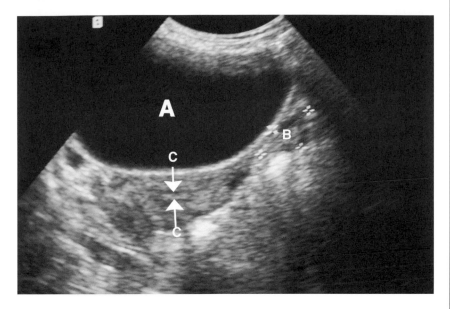

Question 6

1. Name structure A.
2. Name structure B.
3. What are the normal dimensions of structure B in an adult?
4. Name structure C.
5. In the immediate premenstrual period, what is the thickness of C?

Exam 7

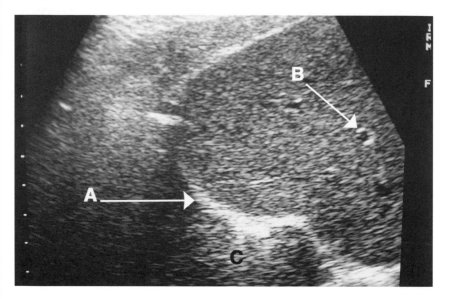

Question 7

1. Name structure A.
2. What frequency transducer should be used for this examination?
3. Name structure B.
4. Give one ultrasound criterion for distinguishing between portal and hepatic veins on ultrasound.
5. What is C and what causes its appearance?

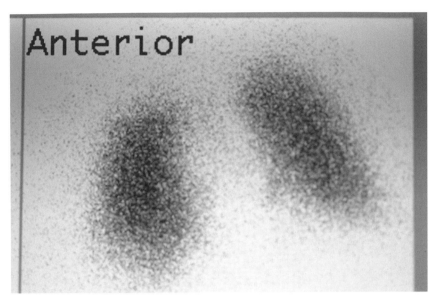

Question 8

1. What investigation is this and what radiopharmaceutical agent has been used?
2. What is the typical dose administered for such a test?
3. What is the normal positioning for this patient and how is the agent routinely administered?
4. What is the normal size of the particles administered?
5. What percentage of the pulmonary bed is typically occluded by the particles?

Exam 7

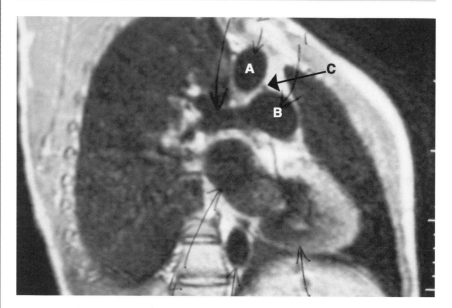

Question 9

1. What investigation is this and what view is shown?
2. Name structure A.
3. Why is structure A of low signal?
4. Name structure B.
5. Name structure C.

Exam 7

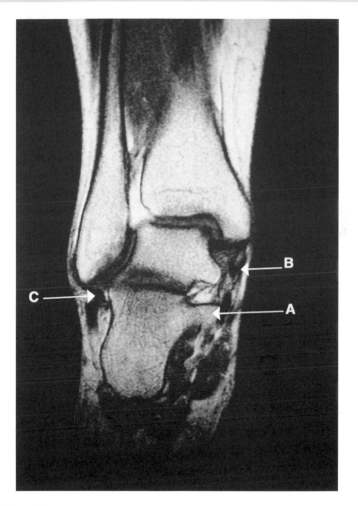

Question 10

1. What imaging sequence is this?
2. Name structure A.
3. Name structure B.
4. Name structure C.
5. What is the Larmor equation?

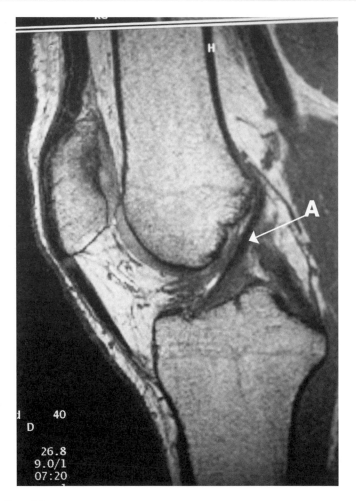

Question 11

1. What is this examination?
2. Name structure A.
3. What is the attachment for A on the femur?
4. Does this image demonstrate a medial or lateral view and how do you know?
5. MR scanners routinely scan from right to left: true or false?

Exam 7

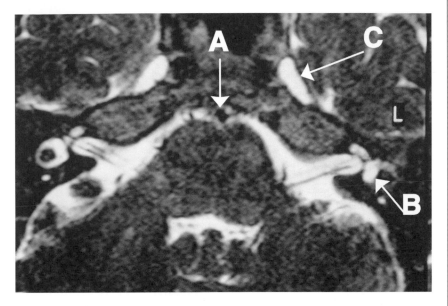

Question 12

1. What sequence and imaging plane has been performed?
2. Name structure A.
3. Name structure B.
4. Name structure C.
5. Why does C have a high signal and what structure does it contain?

Exam 7

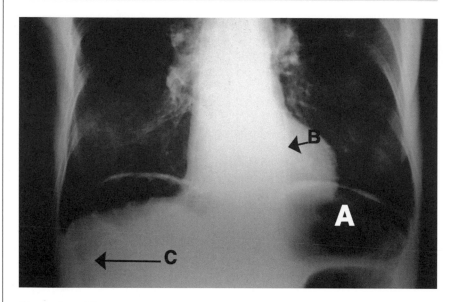

Question 13

1. What is the normal variant shown?
2. Name structure A.
3. What forms line B?
4. At what level does structure B pierce the diaphragm?
5. Name structure C.

Exam 7

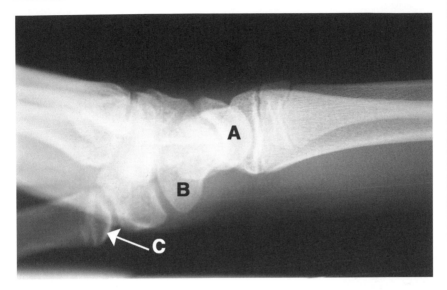

Question 14

1. What is the centering point for this view?
2. Name structure A.
3. Name structure B.
4. Name structure C.
5. How does the location of C differ from that of the other metacarpals?

Exam 7

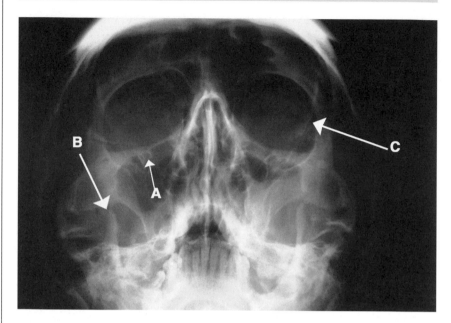

Question 15

1. What view is demonstrated?
2. Name structure A.
3. What structure passes through A?
4. Name structure B.
5. Name structure C.

Exam 7

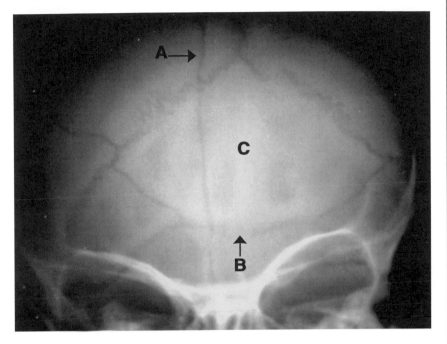

Question 16

1. Name structure A.
2. Name structure B.
3. Name structure C.
4. At what age does structure A fuse?
5. What is the name given to bones lying within sutures?

Exam 7

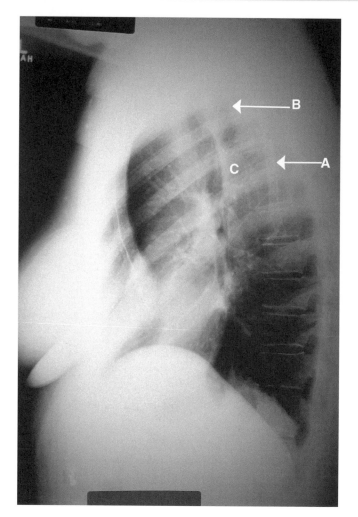

Question 17

1. What is the normal variant shown?
2. Name structure A.
3. Name structure B.
4. Name structure C.
5. What is a centering point for this investigation?

Exam 7

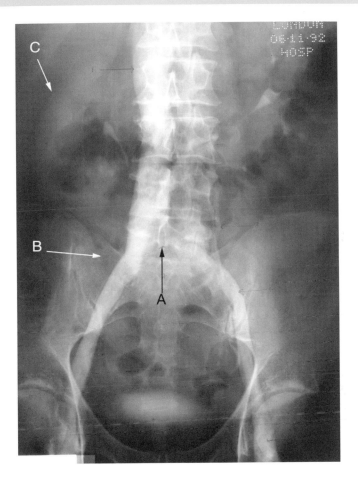

Question 18

1. What is this investigation?
2. Name structure A.
3. Name structure B.
4. Name structure C.
5. Why might the patient be asked to perform a Valsalva manoeuvre during this procedure?

Exam 7

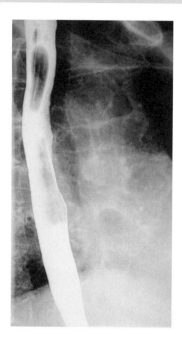

Question 19

1. What is this investigation?
2. What type of barium is commonly used and what is the normal concentration?
3. What view is this?
4. Name two contraindications to the use of barium.
5. What is the optimal patient position to check for gastrooesophageal reflux?

Exam 7

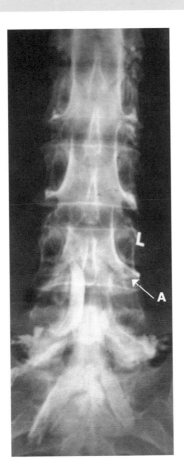

Question 20

1. What is this investigation?
2. Into which dural space is contrast injected?
3. Give two contraindications to this study.
4. Name structure A.
5. At what level does the spinal cord end in (i) adults and (ii) children?

Question 1

1. This is a selective hepatic arteriogram.
2. A = gastroduodenal artery.
3. B = right gastric artery.
4. C = right hepatic artery.
5. The right hepatic artery arises from the SMA in 25% of normal patients.

Question 2

1. A = left internal iliac artery.
2. B = left inferior gluteal artery.
3. C = left iliolumbar artery.
4. D = posterior division of the right internal iliac artery.
5. E = uterine artery.

Question 3

1. This is a digital subtraction vertebral angiogram. A lateral view is demonstrated.
2. Usually only the left vertebral artery needs to be cannulated, as this is usually the dominant artery and reflux into the right vertebral frequently occurs.
3. A = anterior inferior cerebellar artery.
4. B = posterior cerebral artery.
5. C = basilar artery. This lies in the prepontine cistern.

Question 4

1. A = fissure for the ligamentum teres.
2. The umbilical vein runs in structure A.
3. Water is given as an oral contrast agent when imaging the oesophagus, stomach, duodenum and pancreas.
4. Water is a negative contrast agent.
5. B = intrahepatic part of the inferior vena cava.

Question 5

1. A = right foramen transversarium.
2. The right vertebral artery, a branch of the subclavian artery, runs through the foramen transversarium.
3. This is a view of the cervical spine – indicated by the presence of a foramen transversarium and a bifid spinous process.
4. CT has far better contrast resolution compared with plain film radiography and, as a result, less contrast medium is required.
5. B = contrast within the subarachnoid space.

Question 6

1. A = bladder.
2. B = left ovary.
3. The normal dimensions of the ovary in an adult female = $2 \times 3 \times 4$ cm.
4. C = endometrium.
5. The thickness of the endometrium in the immediate premenstrual period = 10–14 mm.

Question 7

1. A = right hemidiaphragm.
2. A 3.5 MHz frequency transducer is routinely used.
3. B = portal venous radical.
4. Portal veins have echogenic walls whilst hepatic veins do not.
5. C = mirror image artefact. This occurs in a region which has a strong reflector, such as the diaphragm. The echoes lying to one side of the strong reflector are interpreted as arising on both sides of it and, as in this example, an image of the liver is produced lying within the lung.

Question 8

1. This is the perfusion part of a ventilation perfusion radionuclide scan (as opposed to the ventilation part of the scan as no tracer is identified within the trachea). The agent administered is ^{99m}Tc–MAA.
2. Administered dose is typically 100 MBq.
3. The agent is administered intravenously with the patient in a supine position.
4. Particle size = 10–100 μm.
5. Typically 0.5% of the pulmonary bed is occluded by the particles.

Question 9

1. This is a coronal oblique MRI of the chest.
2. A = arch of aorta.
3. The arch of aorta is of low signal due to flow void phenomena.
4. B = pulmonary trunk.
5. C = ligamentum arteriosum.

Question 10

1. This is a T1 W coronal section through the ankle.
2. A = sustentaculum tali.
3. B = tendon of flexor hallucis longus.
4. C = tendon of peroneus brevis.
5. Larmor equation: frequency = magnetic field strength $\times$ gyromagnetic ratio.

Question 11

1. This is a T1-weighted sagittal MR of the knee.
2. A = anterior cruciate ligament.
3. The femoral attachment of A = medial aspect of the lateral femoral condyle.
4. This is a medial image of the knee as the fibula is not present.
5. True.

Question 12

1. This is an axial T2-weighted scan.
2. A = basilar artery.
3. B = vestibular part of the left inner ear.
4. C = left Meckel's cave.
5. Meckel's cave is a dural cave containing CSF and houses the trigeminal ganglia.

Question 13

1. The variant demonstrated is Chilaiditi's syndrome. This is caused by a loop of colon interposing between the diaphragm and the superior surface of the liver.
2. A = fundal gas shadow.
3. B = descending thoracic aorta.
4. The descending aorta pierces the diaphragm at T12.
5. C = a haustral fold in the ascending colon/hepatic flexure.

Question 14

1. The centering point is the radial styloid process.
2. A = lunate.
3. B = scaphoid.
4. C = ossification centre (epiphysis) for the first metacarpal.
5. The ossification centre for the first metacarpal is at its base, whereas for the remaining metacarpals the ossification centre is at their distal ends.

Question 15

1. This is an occipitomental view (OM).
2. A = infraorbital foramen.
3. The infraorbital nerve and artery pass through the infraorbital foramen.
4. B = right coronoid process.
5. C = left innominate line.

Question 16

1. A = metopic suture.
2. B = mendosal suture.
3. C = inca bone.
4. The metopic suture fuses at 5 years of age.
5. Bones lying within sutures are known as wormian bones.

Question 17

1. The lower aspect of the sternum is depressed. Diagnosis: pectus excavatum.
2. A = lateral border of the scapula.
3. B = trachea.
4. C = arch of the aorta.
5. The centering point is through the axilla directed to the middle of the film.

Question 18

1. This is an inferior venocavogram.
2. A = spinous process of L5.
3. B = right sacral ala.
4. C = right renal outline.
5. The patient is asked to perform a Valsalva manoeuvre in order to retard the flow of contrast to the thorax and thus maximize opacification of the IVC.

Question 19

1. This is a barium swallow.
2. Baritop; 100% w/v is commonly used.
3. This is an erect view in RAO position.
4. Contraindications to barium: recent gastrointestinal surgery, perforated viscus and aspiration.
5. The patient should be examined in a prone position.

Question 20

1. This is a lumbar myelogram.
2. Contrast is injected into the subarachnoid space.
3. Contraindications:
    (i)   raised intracranial pressure.
    (ii) lumbar puncture in the previous week.
    (iii) previous reaction to intrathecal contrast.
4. A = left L4 nerve root.
5. (i)   In adults the spinal cord ends at L1–2.
   (ii) In children the spinal cord ends at L3–4.

Exam 8

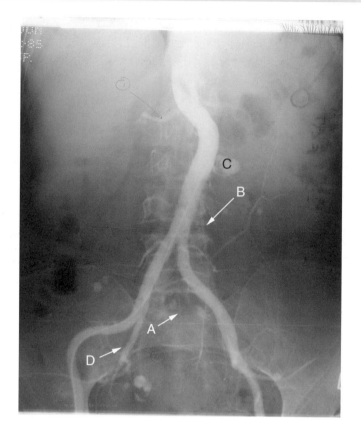

Question 1

1. Name structure A.
2. Name structure B.
3. Name structure C.
4. Name structure D.
5. What are the defining characteristics of:
   (i) Terumo wire?
   (ii) Amplatz guide wire?

Exam 8

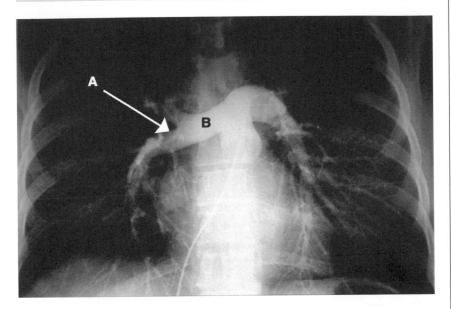

Question 2

1. What investigation is this?
2. What catheter is used and where should it be sited?
3. What volume of contrast is used and what is the rate of infusion?
4. Name structure A.
5. Name structure B and give its relation to the right main bronchus.

Exam 8

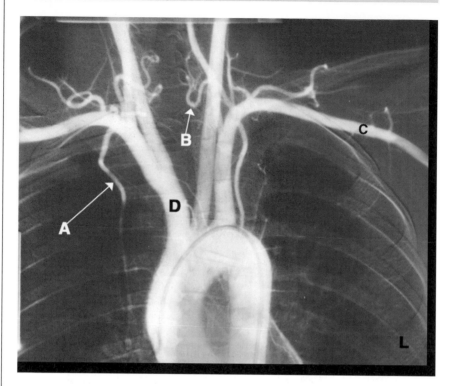

Question 3

1. What is this investigation? How much contrast is given and at what rate?
2. Name structure A.
3. Name structure B.
4. Name structure C.
5. Name structure D.

Exam 8

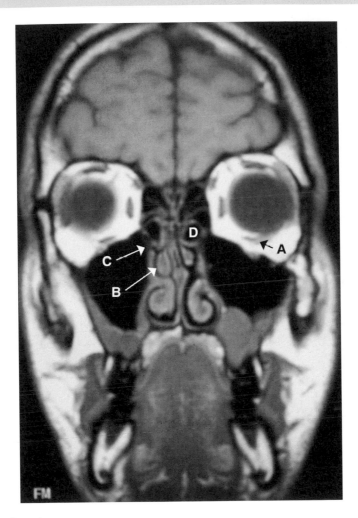

Question 4

1. Name structure A.
2. Name structure B.
3. Name structure C.
4. Name structure D and why does it return a low signal?
5. Why does air return a low signal?

Exam 8

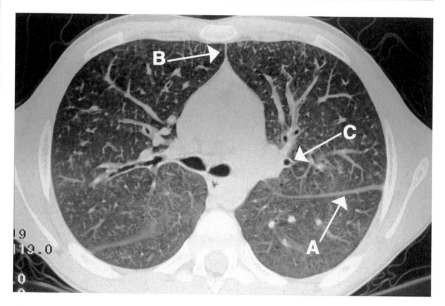

Question 5

1. Name structure A.
2. Name structure B.
3. Name structure C.
4. How can the horizontal fissure be identified on an axial CT scan?
5. Why are patients sometimes turned into a prone position during an HRCT of the chest?

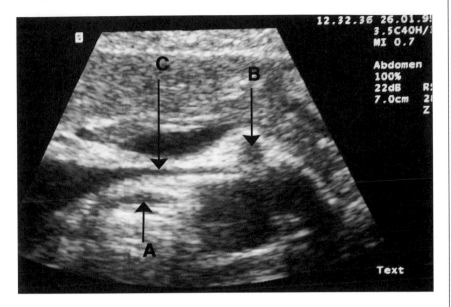

Question 6

1. Name structure A.
2. Name structure B.
3. Name structure C.
4. List the pancreas, kidneys, spleen and liver in decreasing order of echogenicity in a child.
5. What part of the pancreas lies behind structure B?

Exam 8

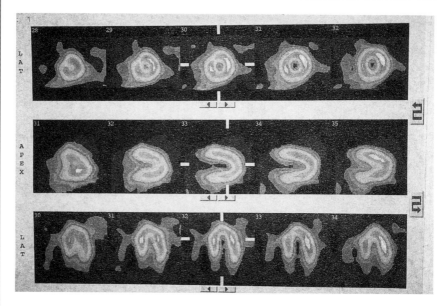

Question 7

1. What is this investigation?
2. Name two radionuclides that can be used for this study.
3. What phases are performed in this test?
4. Provide three methods of inducing a stress within the heart.
5. Which vessel is the main blood supply to the cardiac apex?

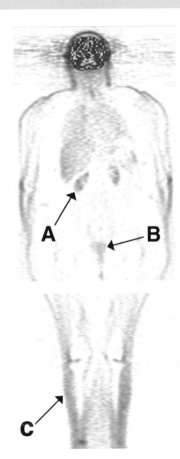

Question 8

1. What is this study?
2. What agent has been used?
3. Name structure A.
4. Name structure B.
5. Name structure C.

Exam 8

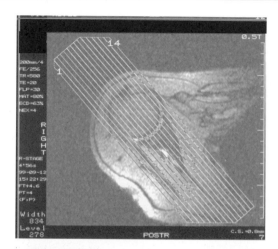

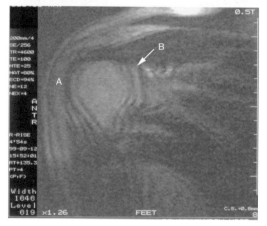

Question 9

1. Why is this study suboptimal?
2. What sequence is this?
3. If the number of phase-encoding steps is 256, what is the scanning time?
   - (i)   230 seconds.
   - (ii)   470 seconds.
   - (iii)   860 seconds.
4. Name structure A.
5. Name structure B.

Exam 8

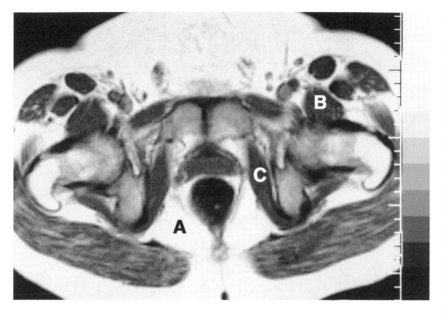

Question 10

1. What sequence has been performed?
2. Name structure A.
3. Name structure B.
4. Name structure C.
5. Is a full bladder essential for pelvic MRI?

Exam 8

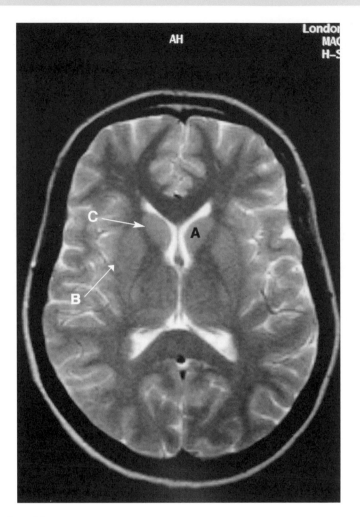

Question 11

1. Name structure A.
2. Name structure B.
3. Name structure C.
4. Name two tissue types that return low signal on both T1 W and T2 W MRI images.
5. Has gadolinium been given for this investigation? Explain why.

Exam 8

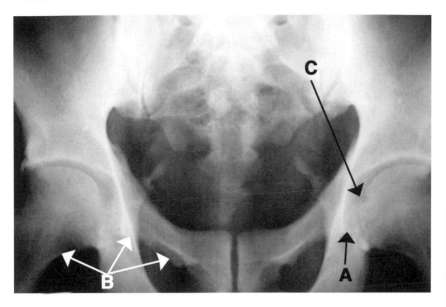

Question 12

1. What is the normal variant shown?
2. Name structure A.
3. Name structure B.
4. What attaches to point C?
5. What is the centering point for:
   (i)   pelvic X-ray?
   (ii)   AP hip X-ray.

Exam 8

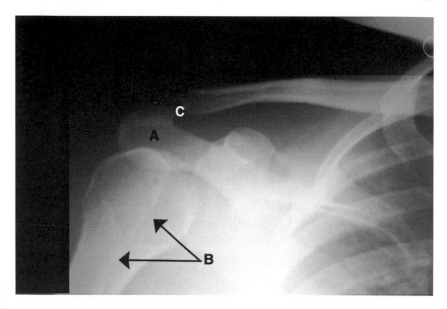

Question 13

1. What is the normal distance A?
2. Which tendons run through A?
3. Name structure B.
4. What is the normal distance C?
5. Give two other views typically performed to image the shoulder.

Exam 8

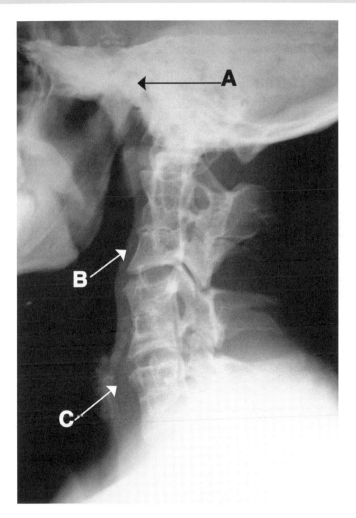

Question 14

1. What is the normal variant shown?
2. What syndrome is this variant often associated with?
3. What is the normal maximum thickness of prevertebral soft tissues at B and C in an adult?
4. Name structure A.
5. How many cervical nerves are there and where do they exit in relation to their vertebra?

Exam 8

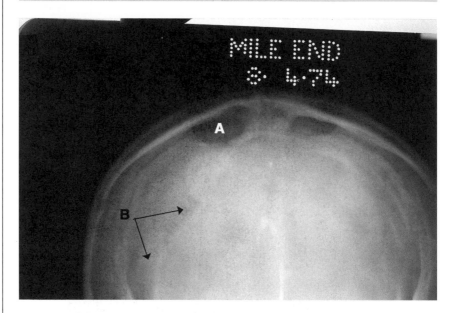

Question 15

1. Name structure A.
2. Which layer(s) of the calvarium does structure A involve?
3. How does structure A differ from a parietal foramen?
4. What view has this image most probably been taken from?
5. Name structure B.

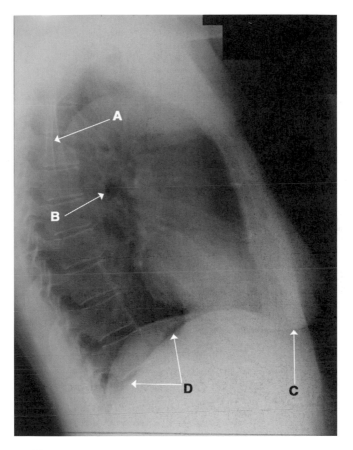

Question 16

1. Name structure A.
2. Name structure B.
3. Name structure C.
4. Name structure D.
5. What are appropriate kVs for a PA and lateral chest X-ray?

Exam 8

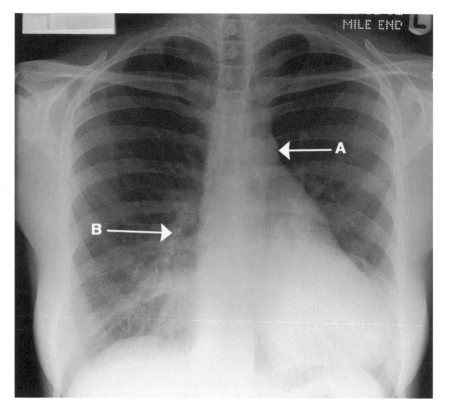

Question 17

1. What is the normal variant shown?
2. Name four radiographic features that confirm the diagnosis.
3. What is the 'normal' relationship of the heart to the midline?
4. Name structure A.
5. Name structure B.

Exam 8

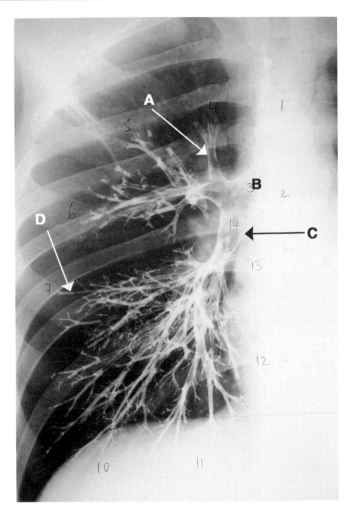

Question 18

1. What is this investigation? Name two indications for it.
2. What contrast medium is used and what is the maximum volume that may be administered?
3. Which side is done first and why?
4. (i) Name structure A.
   (ii) Name structure B.
5. (i) Name structure C.
   (ii) Name structure D.

Exam 8

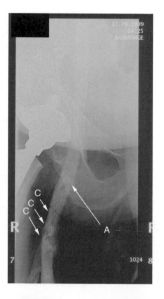

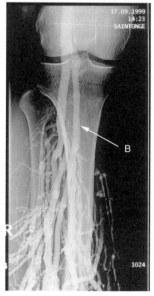

Question 19

1. Name structure A.
2. Name structure B.
3. Name two contraindications to this study.
4. What causes the inhomogeneous opacification at C?
5. Prior to removal of the needle at the end of the study, what should be performed?

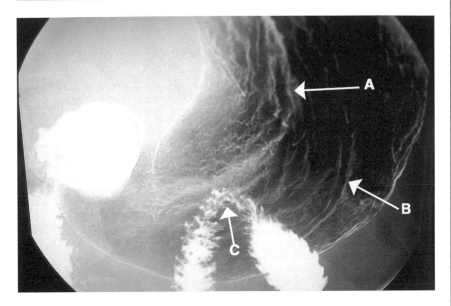

Question 20

1. What position is shown?
2. Name structure A.
3. Name structure B and give its normal thickness.
4. Name structure C.
5. Give three indications for performing a barium meal in children.

Question 1

1. A = median sacral artery.
2. B = inferior mesenteric artery.
3. C = calcified mesenteric lymph node.
4. D = right internal iliac artery.
5. (i) Terumo wire (hydrophilic) – 'slippery wire'.
   (ii) Amplatz wire – 'stiff wire'.

Question 2

1. This is a pulmonary angiogram.
2. A pigtail or NIH catheter may be used for this investigation.
3. 34–40 ml of contrast is used at an infusion rate of 15–20 ml per second.
4. A = interlobar artery (aka right lower lobe artery).
5. B = right pulmonary artery. This lies in front of the right main bronchus.

Question 3

1. This is an arch aortogram. 40 ml of contrast is given at 20 ml per second
2. A = right internal thoracic artery.
3. B = left inferior thyroid artery.
4. C = left axillary artery.
5. D = brachiocephalic trunk.

Question 4

1. A = left inferior rectus muscle.
2. B = right middle concha.
3. C = right osteomeatal complex.
4. D = ethmoid sinus. This returns a low signal as it contains air.
5. Air returns a low signal as it has a minimal hydrogen content.

Question 5

1. A = left oblique fissure.
2. B = anterior junctional line.
3. C = left upper lobe bronchus.
4. On an axial CT scan the horizontal fissure is represented by an avascular plane.
5. In HRCT, patients are turned prone to differentiate between hypostatic change and early fibrosis.

Question 6

1. A = right renal artery.
2. B = SMA.
3. C = left renal vein.
4. Liver, spleen, pancreas and kidneys.
5. The uncinate process lies behind structure B.

Question 7

1. This is a radionuclide myocardial perfusion scan.
2. Radionuclides:
   (i) ^{201}Thallium.
   (ii) ^{99m}Tc-sestamibi.
3. Both resting and stress phases are performed.
4. Stress induction:
   (i)   adenosine.
   (ii)   dipyridamole.
   (iii) exercise.
5. The left anterior descending artery supplies the cardiac apex.

Question 8

1. This is a whole-body positron emission tomogram (PET scan).
2. The agent used is 18-fluorodeoxyglucose (18FDG).
3. A = right kidney.
4. B = bladder.
5. C = muscle activity in the right lower leg.

Question 9

1. There is marked motion artefact.
2. This is a T2-weighted sequence.
3. The total scanning time = TR × NEX × Number of phase encoding steps.
4. A = deltoid muscle.
5. B = superior glenoid labrum.

Question 10

1. This is an axial T1 W MRI of the pelvis.
2. A = right ischioanal fossa.
3. B = left iliopsoas muscle.
4. C = left obturator internus.
5. A full bladder is not essential in pelvic MRI. This is in contradistinction to ultrasound where a full bladder is required to elevate the small bowel loop out of the pelvis.

Question 11

1. A = head of left caudate nucleus.
2. B = right external capsule.
3. C = anterior limb of right internal capsule.
4. Cortical tissue, air and haemosiderin-rich tissue return a low signal on both T1 W and T2 W MRI images.
5. Gadolinium has not been given on this scan. This is a T2 W image, which results in CSF returning high signal.

Question 12

1. Bilateral calcified sacrospinous ligaments are shown.
2. A = Kohler's teardrop.
3. B = Shenton's line.
4. The ligamentum teres attaches to the fovea capitis.
5. Centering points:
   (i) Pelvic X-ray – 5 cm above the superior border of the symphysis pubis.
   (ii) AP hip X-ray – 2.5 cm above the superior border of the symphysis pubis.

Question 13

1. A = acromiohumeral space – 6 mm.
2. The tendons of the rotator cuff and a long head of biceps run through the acromiohumeral space.
3. B = bicipital groove.
4. C = acromioclavicular joint – 7 mm.
5. An axial view and a Y-view are other routinely performed views of the shoulder.

Question 14

1. The variant shown is a fused/blocked cervical vertebra.
2. This is often associated with Klippel–Feil syndrome.
3. B = 7 mm, C = 22 mm.
4. A = mandibular condyle.
5. There are eight cervical nerves. C1–C7 exit above their corresponding vertebra, C8 exits below the C7 vertebra.

Question 15

1. A = pacchonian granulation.
2. The pacchonian granulation involves the inner table only.
3. A parietal foramen affects both layers of the calvarium.
4. This image has been taken from a Towne's view.
5. B = lambdoid suture.

Question 16

1. A = blade of the scapula.
2. B = left main bronchus.
3. C = inferior aspect of breast shadow.
4. D = right hemidiaphragm.
5. PA chest X-ray = 65 kVp, lateral chest X-ray = 75 kVp.

Question 17

1. The normal variant shown is a pectus excavatum.
2. Four radiographic features:
    (i)   The ribs have a '7/reverse 7' configuration.
    (ii) The heart is shifted to the left.
    (iii) The left heart border has a vertical orientation.
    (iv) The posterior ribs are horizontal in orientation and the anterior ribs are more vertical in orientation than normal.
3. Normally two-thirds of the heart is to the left of the midline, whilst one-third is to the right.
4. A = aortic knuckle.
5. B = soft tissue shadow of the interlobar artery.

Question 18

1. This is a bronchogram.
Indications:
    (i)   bronchiectasis.
    (ii) to demonstrate the site and extent of bronchial obstruction.
2. A low osmolar contrast medium is frequently used, e.g. omnipaque. 2–3 ml of contrast is used per lung segment and a maximum of 25 ml may be used per patient.
3. The right side is routinely performed first as a lateral view is only performed on the right side. If the left lung were performed first, the oblique images required on this side would interfere with the right lateral images.
4. (i)   A = apical segment of the right upper lobe.
   (ii) B = right main bronchus.
5. (i)   C = bronchus intermedius.
   (ii) D = lateral segment of the right middle lobe.

Question 19

1. A = great saphenous vein.
2. B = posterior tibial vein.
3. Contraindications: local sepsis and contrast reactions.
4. Flow (streaming) causes the inhomogeneous opacification at C.
5. The line should be flushed with saline to prevent chemical phlebitis.

Question 20

1. The position shown is LAO.
2. A = longitudinal rugae of the 'magenstrassa' parallelling the lesser curve.
3. B = normal gastric rugae – normal thickness 3–5 mm.
4. C = duodenojejunal flexure (ligament of Treitz).
5. Barium meal in children:
    (i)   Assessment of gastrooesophageal reflux.
    (ii) Assessment of malrotation.
    (iii) Investigation of congenital hypertrophic pyloric stenosis.

Exam 9

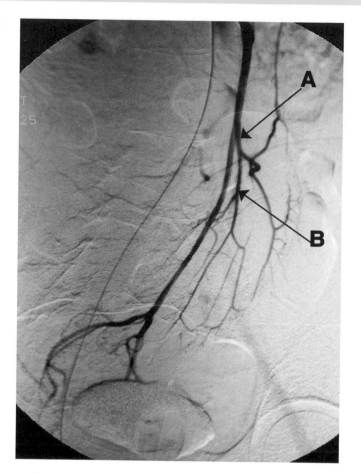

Question 1

1. What is this investigation?
2. At what level is the catheter?
3. Name structure A.
4. Name structure B.
5. Why might this investigation be done first in selective mesenteric angiography?

Exam 9

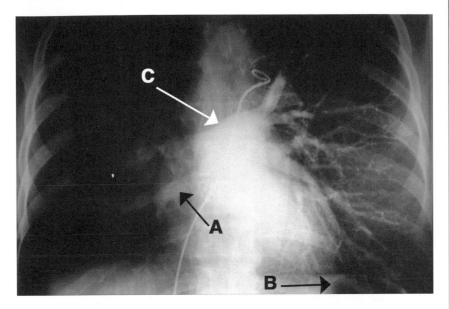

Question 2

1. What is this investigation?
2. In what structure does the catheter lie?
3. Name structure A.
4. Name structure B.
5. Name structure C.

Exam 9

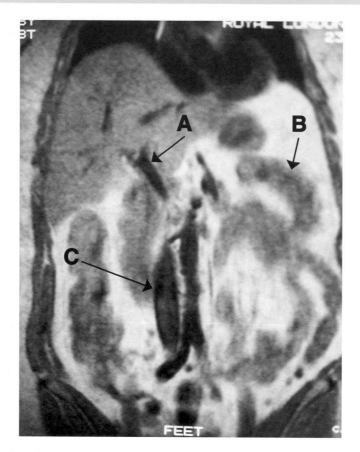

Question 3

1. Name structure A.
2. Name structure B.
3. Name structure C.
4. At what level does structure C begin?
5. Where does the left common iliac vein lie in relation to the right common iliac artery and what sign is attributed to this on a venogram?

Exam 9

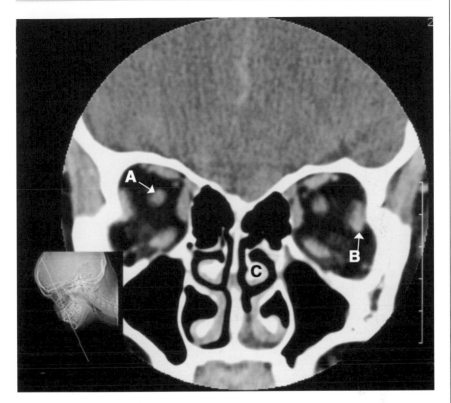

Question 4

1. What is this investigation?
2. Name structure A.
3. Name structure B.
4. Name structure C.
5. How is the patient positioned for this investigation?

Exam 9

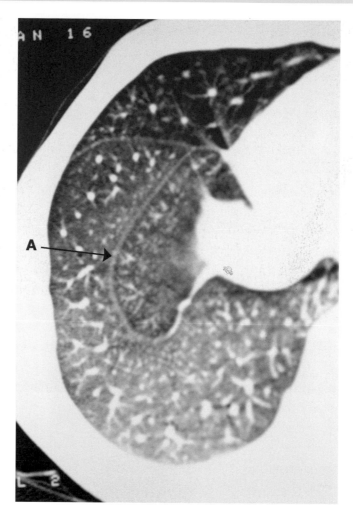

Question 5

1. What type of investigation is this?
2. Name structure A.
3. From how many layers of pleura is structure A formed?
4. What is the normal slice thickness for such an investigation and at what intervals are slices performed?
5. What is a limiting factor for performing this investigation with even thinner slices?

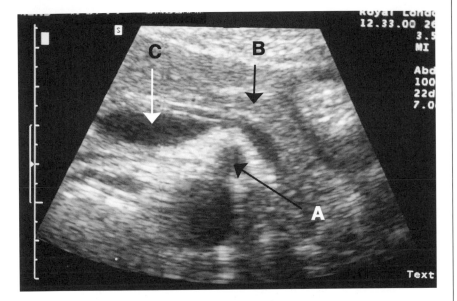

Question 6

1. Name structure A.
2. Name structure B.
3. Name structure C.
4. Name two methods of improving visualization of structure B.
5. What is the purpose of using ultrasound gel?

Exam 9

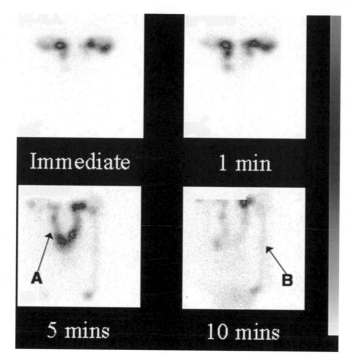

Immediate   1 min

5 mins   10 mins

Question 7

1. What is this investigation?
2. What agent is used?
3. What is the indication?
4. Name structure A.
5. Name structure B.

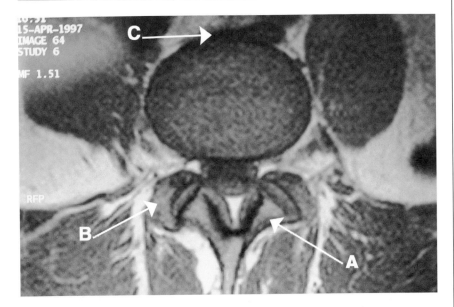

Question 8

1. Name structure A.
2. Name structure B.
3. Name structure C.
4. Give a typical TR and TE for this study.
5. In lumbar spine MRI, what imaging planes and sequences are typically performed?

Exam 9

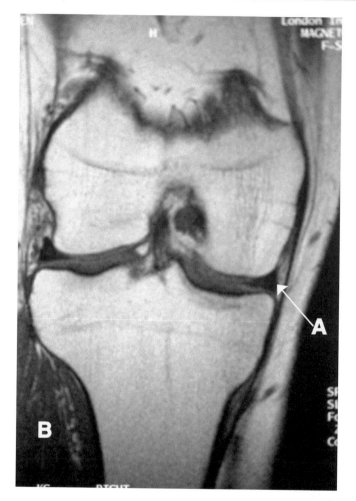

Question 9

1. What imaging sequence has been performed?
2. Name structure A.
3. Name structure B.
4. Name the coolants used in a superconducting magnet.
5. What does the term 'quenching' mean?

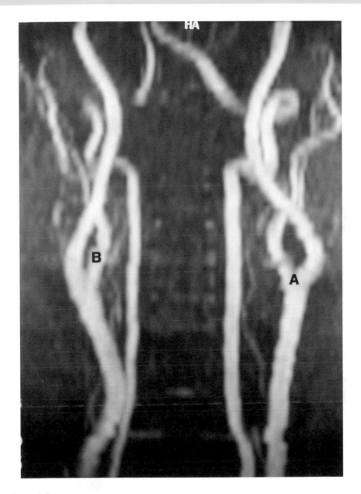

Question 10

1. What is this investigation?
2. What two techniques may be used to perform this study?
3. Name structure A.
4. At what level does structure A typically lie?
5. What is the first branch of structure B?

Exam 9

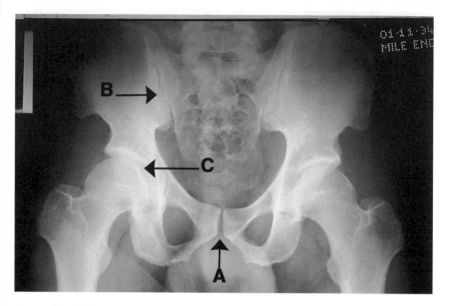

Question 11

1. What type of joint is A?
2. What type of joint is B?
3. What type of joint is C?
4. Describe two methods of performing pelvimetry.
5. Which of these two methods of pelvimetry offers a lower exposure dose to the patient?

Exam 9

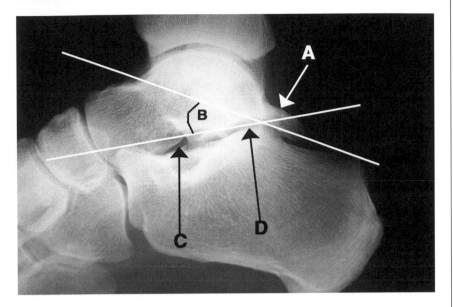

Question 12

1. Name structure A.
2. What is angle B known as?
3. What is the normal range for B?
4. What space does C denote?
5. Name structure D.

Exam 9

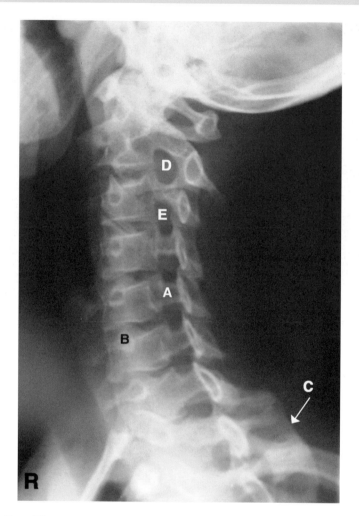

Question 13

1. Name structure A.
2. Name structure B.
3. Name structure C.
4. Name structure D
5. If this is an anterior oblique view, which nerve exits through E?

Exam 9

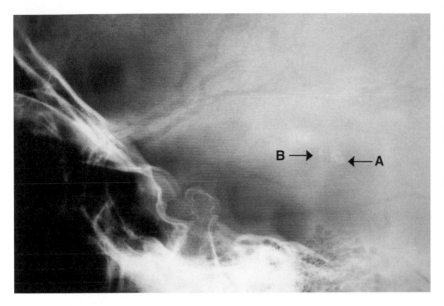

Question 14

1. Name structure A.
2. Name structure B.
3. What is the maximum size of structure A?
4. What is the maximum allowable shift from the midline, for an AP film, for structure A?
5. What is the incidence of A?

Exam 9

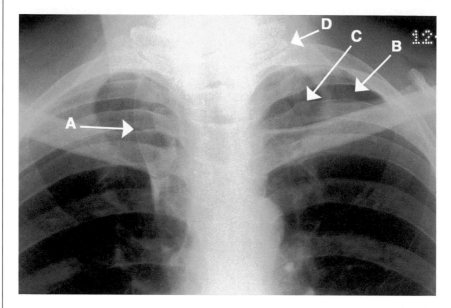

Question 15

1. Name structure A.
2. Name structure B.
3. How is rotation of the patient relative to the film assessed? Comment on the rotation in this image.
4. Name structure C.
5. Name structure D.

Exam 9

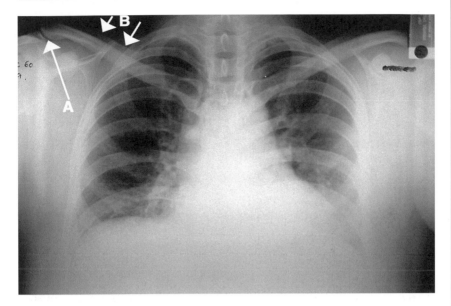

Question 16

1. What is the major technical problem with this film?
2. Which joint is indicated by A and what is its normal width?
3. How do you assess for alignment at this joint?
4. Name structure B.
5. What is the normal interpedicular distance in the adult thoracic spine?

Exam 9

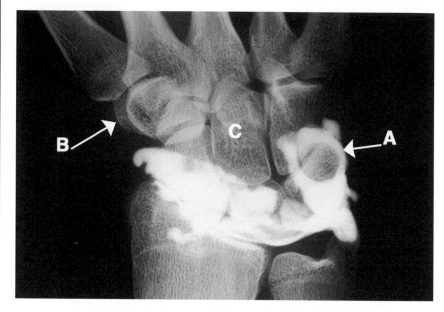

Question 17

1. Name structure A. Is this area usually filled with contrast in a normal arthrogram?
2. Name one contraindication to this study.
3. Name structure B.
4. Name structure C.
5. Are the midcarpal joints normally seen on a wrist arthrogram? Explain your answer.

Exam 9

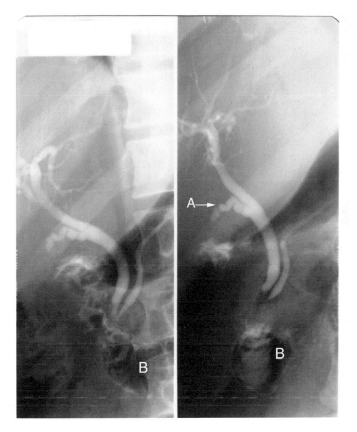

Question 18

1. What is this investigation?
2. Give two reasons why this investigation is *not* a percutaneous trans-hepatic cholangiogram (PTC).
3. Name structure A.
4. Name structure B.
5. What operation has this patient previously undergone?

Exam 9

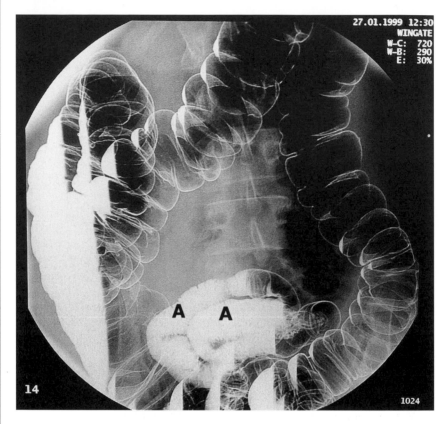

27.01.1999 12:30
WINGATE
W-C: 720
W-B: 290
E: 30%

14

1024

Question 19

1. Give two contraindications to this study.
2. Give three complications that may arise as a result of this investigation.
3. Name structure A.
4. Which views optimally visualize the following:
   (i) sigmoid colon?
   (ii) splenic flexure?
5. Which structure maintains the position of the splenic flexure?

Exam 9

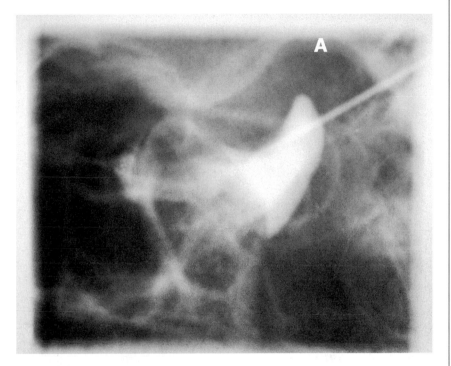

Question 20

1. What is this investigation?
2. Which compartment has contrast been injected into?
3. What volume of contrast is used for this investigation?
4. What views are normally taken?
5. Name structure A.

Question 1

1. This is a selective inferior mesenteric arteriogram.
2. The catheter is at L3.
3. A = left colic artery.
4. B = sigmoid artery.
5. If coeliac or SMA angiography were performed first, contrast would accumulate in the bladder and obscure branches of the IMA within the pelvis. Hence, IMA angiography is performed first.

Question 2

1. This is a venous phase of a pulmonary angiogram.
2. The catheter is situated in the pulmonary trunk.
3. A = right inferior pulmonary vein.
4. B = gas in the fundus of the stomach.
5. C = confluence of the pulmonary vein at the left atrium.

Question 3

1. A = portal vein.
2. B = loop of jejunum.
3. C = IVC.
4. The IVC begins at L5.
5. The left common iliac vein lies behind the right common iliac artery. This is known as the Cockett-Lea-Thomas sign (this appears as a filling defect in the left common iliac vein).

Question 4

1. This is a coronal CT scan of the paranasal sinuses.
2. A = right optic nerve.
3. B = left lateral rectus muscle.
4. C = left middle turbinate.
5. Patient positioning: the patient lies prone with the neck in extension. The CT gantry is tilted prior to scanning.

Question 5

1. This is a HRCT of the chest.
2. A = right inferior accessory fissure.
3. The inferior accessory fissure is formed from two layers of pleura.
4. HRCT: slice thickness = 2 mm, interval between slices = 10–15 mm.
5. If slices less than 2 mm are used, there is an increase in noise which reduces the signal-to-noise ratio.

Question 6

1. A = SMA.
2. B = body of the pancreas.
3. C = portosplenic confluence.
4. Methods for improving visualization of the pancreas include standing the patient erect and using the stomach as an acoustic window following the intake of water.
5. The purpose of the ultrasound gel is to improve the matching of the acoustic impedances between the probe and the patient's skin.

Question 7

1. This is a lacrimal scintogram.
2. Agent: ^{99m}Tc-pertechnetate.
3. Indication: epiphora.
4. A = right nasolacrimal duct.
5. B = artefact caused by tears overflowing the left cheek.

Question 8

1. A = left lamina.
2. B = right superior articular process of the vertebral body above.
3. C = anterior longitudinal ligament.
4. TR = approximately 500–600.
   TE = approximately 20–30.
5. Lumbar spine MRI: sagittal T1 and T2, axial T1 +/- gadolinium.

Question 9

1. This is a coronal T1-weighted image of the knee.
2. A = medial meniscus.
3. B = tibialis anterior muscle.
4. Liquid helium and liquid nitrogen are the coolants used in a super-conducting magnet.
5. The coolant levels must be logged daily. If they fall too low, 'quenching' occurs; the temperature rises, superconductivity is lost and the stored energy is released. If the temperature rises, the liquid gases boil off rapidly and must be vented outside the building.

Question 10

1. This is an MRA of the great vessels in the neck.
2. The two techniques used for this investigation are 2D/3D time-of-flight angiography and phase-contrast angiography.
3. A = left carotid bifurcation.
4. The carotid bifurcation usually lies at C4.
5. B = right external carotid artery. Its first branch is the superior thyroid artery.

Question 11

1. A = symphysis pubis – primary cartilaginous type.
2. B = sacroiliac joint – synovial type.
3. C = hip joint – synovial type.
4. Pelvimetry: plain radiography and CT.
5. CT offers a lower patient dose as compared with plain film radiography.

Question 12

1. A = fused os trigonum.
2. B = Bohler's angle.
3. The normal Bohler's angle = 28–40°.
4. C = sinus tarsi.
5. D = posterior subtalar joint.

Question 13

1. A = lamina of C5.
2. B = transverse process of C6.
3. C = left first rib.
4. D = intervertebral foramina of C2–3.
5. The left C4 nerve root exits through the intervertebral foramen marked E.

Question 14

1. A = calcified pineal gland.
2. B = calcified habenular commissure.
3. The maximum size of structure A = 10 mm.
4. 3 mm is the maximum allowable shift from the midline for the pineal gland.
5. Calcification of the pineal gland occurs in 70% of those over 70 years of age and in only 5% of those less than 10 years of age.

Question 15

1. A = azygous fissure.
2. B = left 1st rib.
3. The spinous processes of the 3rd and 4th thoracic vertebrae should be equally distant from the medial ends of the clavicle when the patient has been positioned correctly. In this image there is slight rotation to the left.
4. C = non-articular tubercle of the left 4th rib.
5. D = costotransverse joint of the left 2nd rib.

Question 16

1. This film is taken in expiration, resulting in apparent cardiomegaly and widening of the superior mediastinum.
2. A = right acromioclavicular joint. Normal width = 7 mm.
3. The acromioclavicular joint is in alignment if the inferior surfaces are continuous with one another.
4. B = companion shadow to the right clavicle.
5. The normal interpedicular distance in the thoracic spine = 20–30 mm.

Question 17

1. A = pisiform recess. This is not seen in a normal arthrogram.
2. Contraindication: local sepsis.
3. B = trapezium.
4. C = capitate.
5. The midcarpal joints are not normally seen as the scapholunate and lunotriquetral ligaments inhibit the flow of contrast.

Question 18

1. This is an ERCP (endoscopic retrograde cholangiopancreatogram).
2. The reasons why this investigation is not a PTC are:
   (i)   no percutaneous needle is seen.
   (ii) the pancreatic duct is identified.
3. A = cystic duct.
4. B = 3rd part of duodenum.
5. This patient has had a cholecystectomy.

Question 19

1. Contraindications: toxic megacolon, pseudomembranous colitis, rectal biopsy via a rigid sigmoidoscope within the preceding 7 days.
2. Complications: bowel perforation, venous extravasation, water intoxication, intramural barium, drug reactions, arrhythmias and bacteraemia.
3. A relates to reflux of contrast into the small bowel.
4. Positions:
   (i)   Sigmoid colon: prone caudal angled tube (Hampton's view).
   (ii) Splenic flexure: erect LAO.
5. The phrenicocolic ligament attaches the splenic flexure to the diaphragm.

Question 20

1. This is a temporomandibular joint (TMJ) arthrogram.
2. Contrast has been injected into the inferior joint space.
3. 0.3–0.6 ml of contrast is used for a TMJ arthrogram.
4. A lateral oblique with the mouth in both open and closed positions is routinely performed.
5. A = mandibular fossa (for articulation with the condylar process of the mandible).

Exam 10

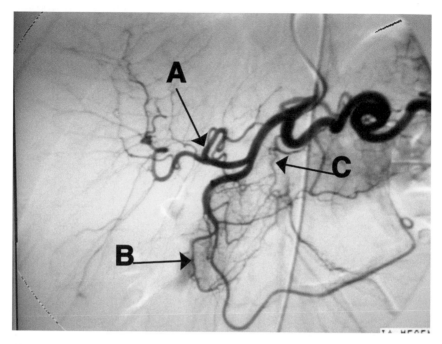

Question 1

1. What is this investigation?
2. Name structure A.
3. Name structure B.
4. Name structure C.
5. What is the approximate infusion rate of contrast used in this investigation?

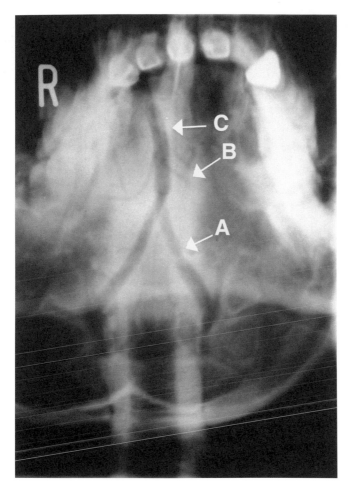

Question 2

1. Name structure A.
2. Name structure B.
3. Name structure C.
4. At what level does the vertebral artery enter the cervical canal?
5. What artery does the posterior inferior cerebellar artery arise from?

Exam 10

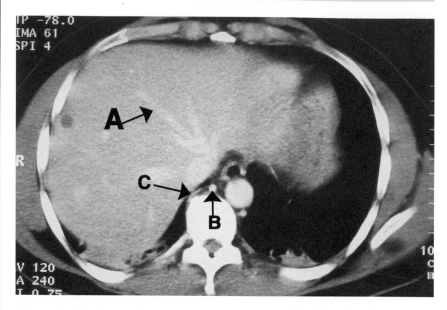

Question 3

1. Name structure A.
2. Name structure B.
3. Name structure C.
4. At what vertebral level does structure B enter the superior vena cava?
5. At what phase of scanning has this scan been performed?

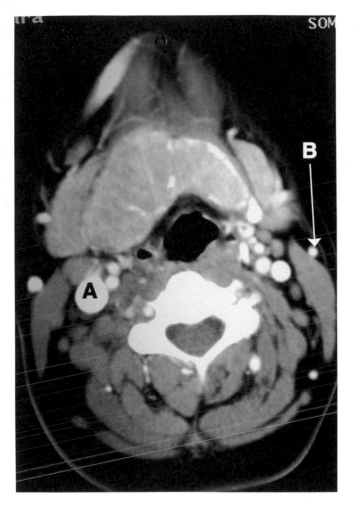

Question 4

1. What normal variant is shown?
2. Name structure A.
3. How does structure A enter the skull?
4. Name structure B.
5. Into what vessel does structure B drain?

Exam 10

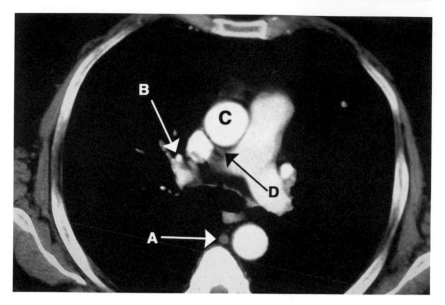

Question 5

1. (i)   Name structure A.
    (ii) Where does it pierce the diaphragm?
2. Name structure B.
3. Name structure C.
4. Name structure D.
5. Define the term 'pitch' as used in helical scanning.

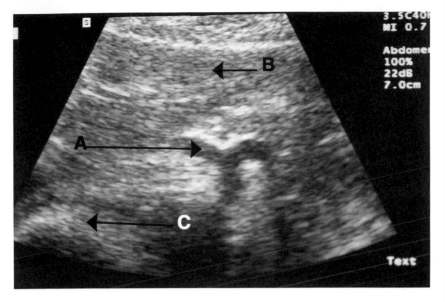

Question 6

1. In which plane has this structure been imaged?
2. At what vertebral level does this structure appear?
3. Name structure A.
4. Name structure B.
5. Name structure C.

Exam 10

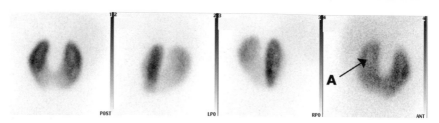

POST   LPO   RPO   ANT

Question 7

1. What is this investigation?
2. What normal variant is demonstrated?
3. What is the incidence of this normal variant?
4. What does A indicate?
5. Why should imaging in the first hour following injection be avoided?

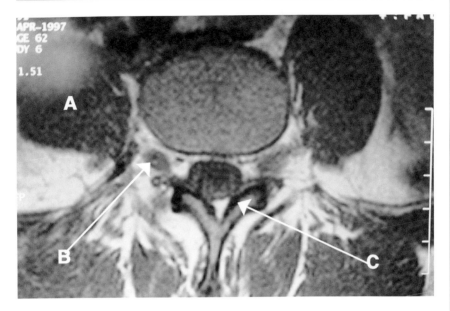

Question 8

1. What is this investigation?
2. Name structure A.
3. Name structure B.
4. What ligament is found at C?
5. Are T1- or T2-weighted images used for gadolinium-enhanced scans and why?

Exam 10

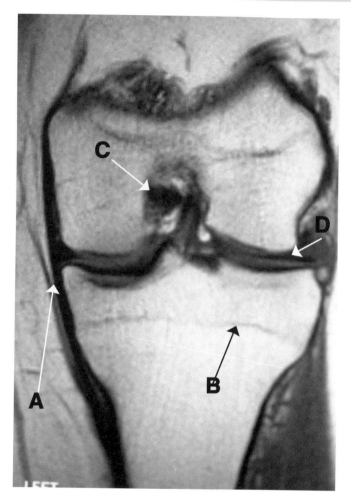

Question 9

1. Name structure A.
2. Name structure B.
3. Name structure C.
4. To image structure C, what sequence and imaging plane is routinely acquired?
5. Name a structure that attaches to D.

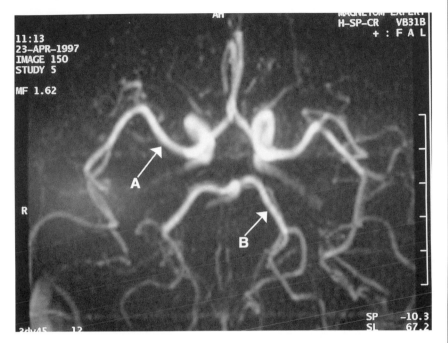

Question 10

1. What is this investigation?
2. Name structure A.
3. Name structure B.
4. Is gadolinium used for this investigation?
5. How is this image formed from individual slices?

Exam 10

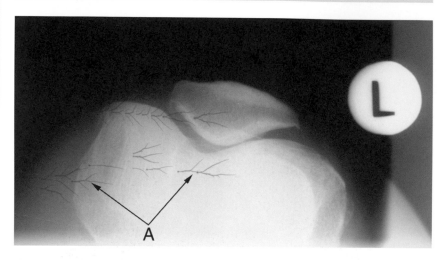

Question 11

1. What view is demonstrated?
2. What is the centering point for this X-ray?
3. What is the cause of the markings labelled A?
4. Is this a routine view for a knee?
5. Which joint is demonstrated and what type of joint is it?

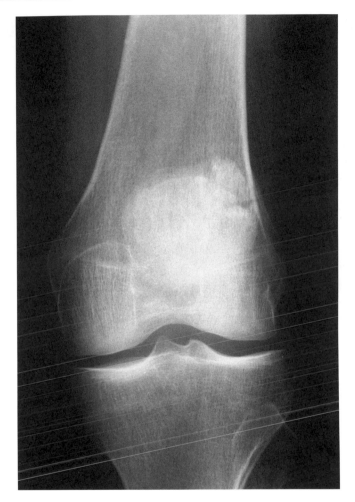

Question 12

1. What normal variant is demonstrated?
2. In which gender is it more common?
3. Is this a more typical site for this variant?
4. How can the patella be better visualised on plain film radiography?
5. What muscles attach to the patella?

Exam 10

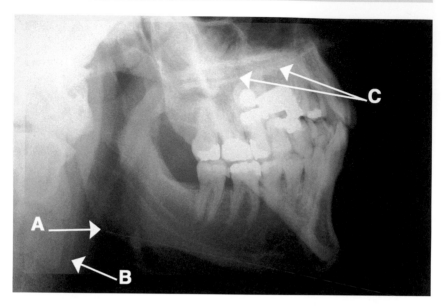

Question 13

1. Name structure A.
2. Name structure B.
3. Name structure C.
4. Give a typical kV for this radiograph.
5. What view is demonstrated?

Exam 10

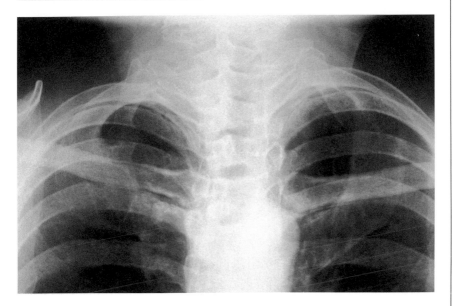

Question 14

1. What is the normal variant shown?
2. Explain the answer to question 1.
3. What is the incidence of this variant?
4. In which sex is this variant more common?
5. In roughly what percentage of cases does this variant occur bilaterally?

Exam 10

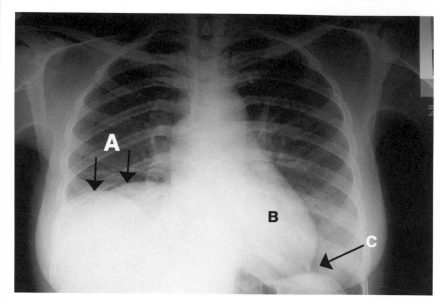

Question 15

1. Name structure A.
2. Why is A normally higher than its counterpart on the left?
3. How should the adequacy of inspiration be assessed on a PA chest X-ray?
4. Which heart chamber is identified by B?
5. Name structure C.

Exam 10

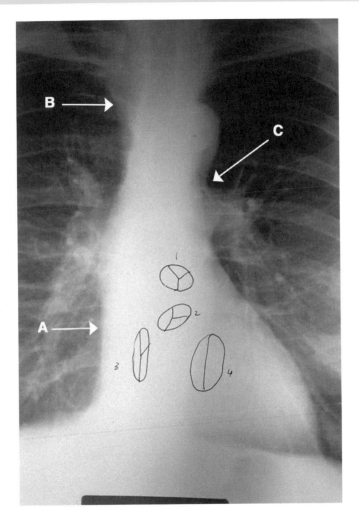

Question 16

1. Name valves 1 and 2.
2. Names valves 3 and 4.
3. Which heart chamber is identified by structure A?
4. Name structure B.
5. Name structure C.

Exam 10

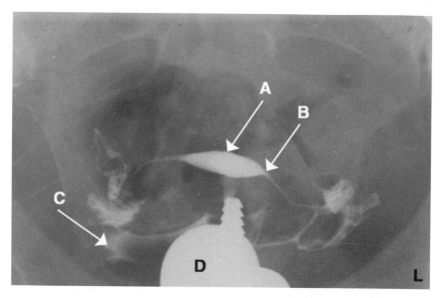

Question 17

1. What is this investigation and what cannula has been used?
2. Name the common indications and two contraindications for this investigation.
3. What is the routine patient preparation prior to this test?
4. Name structures A and B.
5. Name structures C and D.

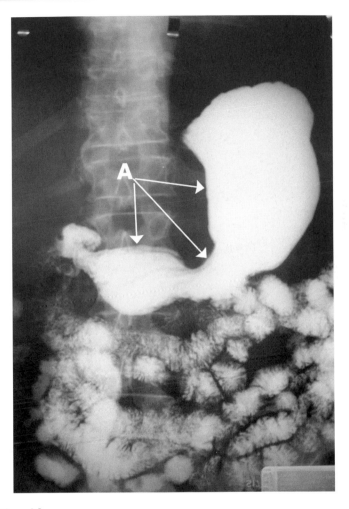

Question 18

1. What is this investigation?
2. Name one other contrast investigation for studying the small bowel.
3. What are the normal maximum dimensions for the following in this investigation:
   (i)   jejunum?
   (ii) terminal ileum?
   (iii) ileal mucosal fold thickness?
4. Name structure A.
5. At what vertebral level does the duodenojejunal flexure normally lie?

Exam 10

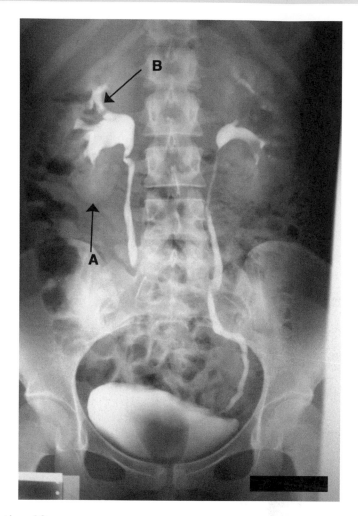

Question 19

1. At what stage in an IVU sequence has this film been taken?
2. Name structure A.
3. Name structure B.
4. What causes the filling defect within the bladder?
5. Give two contraindications to abdominal compression in an IVU.

Exam 10

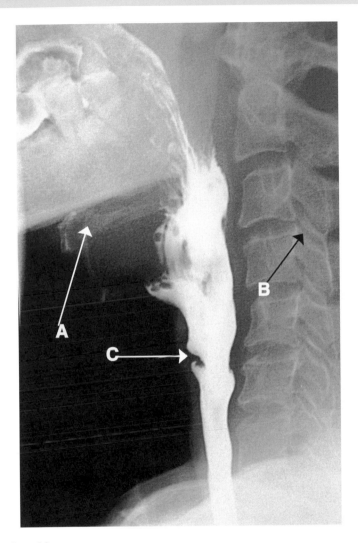

Question 20

1. Name structure A.
2. Name structure B.
3. Name structure C.
4. How would this view be obtained?
5. Name an alternative to barium for a swallow study.

Question 1

1. This is a selective coeliac arteriogram.
2. A = left hepatic artery.
3. B = superior pancreaticoduodenal artery.
4. C = dorsal pancreatic artery.
5. 36 ml of contrast infused at 6 ml per second would be appropriate for this investigation.

Question 2

1. A = left vertebral artery.
2. B = left anterior inferior cerebellar artery.
3. C = basilar artery.
4. In 90% of the population, the vertebral artery enters the cervical canal at C6.
5. The posterior inferior cerebellar artery arises from the vertebral artery.

Question 3

1. A = middle hepatic vein.
2. B = azygous vein.
3. C = right crus of diaphragm.
4. The azygous vein drains into the SVC at T4.
5. This scan has been performed in the portovenous phase.

Question 4

1. The normal variant shown is a lingual thyroid.
2. A = right internal jugular vein.
3. The internal jugular vein enters the skull through the jugular foramen.
4. B = left external jugular vein.
5. The left external jugular veins drains into the left subclavian vein.

Question 5

1. (i)   A = azygous vein.
   (ii)   The azygous vein pierces the diaphragm at T12.
2. B = right superior pulmonary vein.
3. C = ascending aorta.
4. D = superior pericardial recess.
5. Pitch = table movement in one rotation divided by slice thickness (or collimation).

Question 6

1. This is a transverse image of the coeliac artery.
2. The coeliac artery arises at the level of T12.
3. A = common hepatic artery.
4. B = left lobe of the liver.
5. C = vertebral body.

Question 7

1. This is a static DMSA scintigram.
2. A horseshoe kidney is demonstrated.
3. Incidence = 1:400.
4. A indicates a photon-deficient area in the right renal pelvis.
5. Imaging in the first hour is to be avoided because of free ^{99m}Tc in the urine.

Question 8

1. This is a T1 W axial MRI of the lumbar spine.
2. A = right psoas muscle.
3. B = right dorsal root ganglion.
4. The ligamentum flavum lies at C.
5. T1-weighted images are used for gadolinium-enhanced scans. This shortens the longitudinal relaxation time and hence increases the signal from areas of increased uptake.

Question 9

1. A = medial collateral ligament.
2. B = proximal epiphyseal line of the tibia.
3. C = posterior cruciate ligament.
4. For optimal imaging of C; sagittal oblique volume sequence, T1 W.
5. D = lateral meniscus; the popliteus tendon is attached to this.

Question 10

1. This is an MRA of the circle of Willis.
2. A = right middle cerebral artery.
3. B = left posterior cerebral artery.
4. Gadolinium is not routinely used in this investigation.
5. Maximum intensity projection (MIP) is used to form an image from individual slices.

Question 11

1. This is an axial (skyline) view of the patella.
2. Centering point:
   Patient position: patient seated on the examination table. Leg flexed to about 60°. Patella parallel to the table. Cassette placed upright on the thigh perpendicular to the table. Upper border of cassette is one hand's breadth above the patella.
   Central ray: directed to the midpoint of the lower border of the patella, perpendicular to the middle of the cassette.
3. A is caused by a static artefact.
4. This is not a routine view of the knee.
5. The left patellofemoral joint is demonstrated. It is a synovial joint.

Question 12

1. A bipartite patella is demonstrated.
2. This variant is much more common in men.
3. This is a typical appearance for this variant – usually the upper and outer aspect is bipartite.
4. Axial/skyline views will provide better visualization of the patella.
5. The vastus medialis, intermedius, lateralis and rectus femoris muscles attach to the patella.

Question 13

1. A = angle of the mandible.
2. B = prevertebral soft tissue.
3. C = hard palate.
4. A typical kV for this radiograph = 60 kV.
5. This is a lateral oblique of the mandible and not a lateral view of the mandible, as both mandibles do not overlap.

Question 14

1. Bilateral cervical ribs are shown.
2. The transverse processes of cervical ribs are orientated in a caudal direction. Compare this with thoracic transverse processes with a cranial orientation.
3. The incidence of cervical ribs = 1%.
4. Cervical ribs are more common in females.
5. In approximately 50% of cases, cervical ribs occur bilaterally.

Question 15

1. A = diaphragmatic hump of the right hemidiaphragm.
2. The right hemidiaphragm is normally higher than the left due to the underlying upward pressure from the liver.
3. There has been adequate inspiration on a PA chest X-ray if six anterior ribs or 10 posterior ribs are visible in the midclavicular line.
4. B = right ventricle.
5. C = left cardiophrenic angle.

Question 16

1. Valve 1 = pulmonary valve.
   Valve 2 = aortic valve.
2. Valve 3 = tricuspid valve.
   Valve 4 = mitral valve.
3. A = right atrium.
4. B = right lateral border of the manubrium sternum.
5. C = aortopulmonary window.

Question 17

1. This is a hysterosalpingogram. A Leech–Wilkinson cannula has been used.
2. The common indications include infertility, recurrent miscarriages and following tubal surgery. Contraindications include pregnancy, a purulent discharge on inspection of the vulva or cervix and recent dilatation and curettage, abortion or immediately postmenstruation.
3. Patient preparation: the examination should be booked between the 4th and 10th days in a patient with a regular 28-day menstrual cycle. This reduces the risk of intravasation of contrast during the procedure.
4. A = body of uterus, B = left cornu of uterus.
5. C = peritoneal spill of contrast, D = speculum.

Question 18

1. This is an image from a barium follow-through sequence.
2. Alternatively the small bowel may be imaged via a small bowel enema/enteroclysis.
3. Dimensions:
   (i)   Jejunum – 3.5 cm.
   (ii) Terminal ileum – 2 cm.
   (iii) Ileal mucosal fold thickness – 2 mm.
4. A = lesser curvature of the stomach.
5. The DJ flexure normally lies to the left of L2.

Question 19

1. This is a release film in an IVU sequence.
2. A = lower pole of right kidney.
3. B = infundibulum to right upper pole calyx.
4. The lucent filling defect within the bladder is caused by gas within the rectum.
5. Contraindications to abdominal compression:
     (i)   recent abdominal surgery.
     (ii) abdominal aortic aneurysm.
     (iii) presence of a stoma.
     (iv) renal obstruction.
     (v)   pelvic kidneys.
     (vi) after renal trauma.
     (vii) large abdominal mass.

Question 20

1. A = greater cornua of the hyoid bone.
2. B = facet joint C3–4.
3. C = postcricoid venous plexus.
4. This is a lateral view with rapid-sequence radiography.
5. Gastromiro or Omnipaque may be used instead of barium.

NOTES

NOTES

NOTES

NOTES